As a breast cancer physici[...]
to all cancer patients. It i[...]
could read only the parts t[...] [...] come
back and read other parts later. Of most help, are the specific actions patients can - and should - do to help themselves through the cancer journey.

Dr. Robyn Young, MD Medical Oncologist

Doctors are mostly focused on the medical treatment of cancer and may not have the time to explore the very essential emotional aspect. Dr. Barr offers thoughtful, practical tips to patients with newly diagnosed or recurrent cancer, in different stages of treatment.

Dr. Prasanthi Ganesa, MD Medical Oncologist

As a Breast cancer survivor and a cancer Clinician, I was very interested in this book for both my patients and myself. It is so important to have well written and easy to understand resources available to us.

Helena Iannaccone, Oncology Nurse Practitioner

Dr. Niki Barr's book is that unique book that bridges the gap of a cancer diagnosis from the physical to the emotional. It is a 'how to' book on emotional survival; not just for the patient, but, caregiver, partner and maily member. Dr. Barr's 'healing tools' are invaluable. While the surgeon can remove the cancer, recovering from the emotional challenges can be successful with the guidance from this book.

Katherine Stephens, Breast Cancer Survivor and Breast Health Advocate

On behalf of the patient community I have to say "Thank you Niki Barr!" Finally, we have a brillant resource for handling cancer's emotional battlefront. Let the medical community deal with your physical health and let Niki Barr, PhD put you back in charge of your life."

Jim Skinner, Cancer Survivor and Host of Stories With A Purpose

Emotions continually impact patients, survivors, family members and caregivers coping with cancer. Dr. Barr's new book powerfully addresses these emotions, providing needed strategies for amplifying emotional wellbeing.

Lori Drew, Director External Relations, Cancer Treatment Center

Working side by side with Dr. Barr was always an inspiration. I loved seeing the patients and family members who met with her unwind and gradually stand tall. Empowerment, empathy and encouragement is now available for all who read this book!

Valerie Oxford, MSSW, Social Work Supervisor Cancer Treatment Center

In her new book, author and clinician Niki Barr, Ph.D. has given us an actionable roadmap along the emotional collision course called cancer. I highly recommend this book to anyone who has been diagnosed with cancer and also to those who love and care for them.

Sheri Hendricks , Cancer Patient Advocate, Navigator, and Coach

This book includes practical and helpful tips for the cancer patient, family, and friends to survive the cancer journey with emotional wellness. Easy to understand ways to handle emotions and where to turn for added support. Niki has taken the best advice from her years of therapy with cancer patients and their caregivers and put it all together in this book.

Jane Oderberg,Chief Program Officer/Social Worker Cancer Resource Center

Cancer is a forever chapter in your life.

Niki Barr

Given that cancer is a forever chapter, the challenge becomes incorporating the lived experience into who you are rather than allowing the cancer to define who you are. In Getting Off the Emotional Roller Coaster of Cancer, Barr encourages each of us to ask the deeper questions so that we can lay hold of emotional health and wellbeing as we live beyond cancer while providing a multitude of tools to assist us as we navigate those 'in the moment' emotions that can, at times, become overwhelming. Here's to approaching 'the rest of the story' readily equipped to handle whatever come what may.

Stephanie Zimmerman, MSN
Young Adult Survivor of Childhood Cancer and Heart Recipient

In "Getting Off the Emotional Roller Coaster of Cancer" Dr. Niki Barr combines her vast clinical knowledge with her deep compassion for cancer patients and their caregivers. This book is a must for those navigating this most difficult terrain.

Jennifer Warden, M.S.S.A.

Empathic. Informative. This must read book provides coping tools to all who are touched by cancer.

Mary Orndorff, LCSW, LMFT, Psychotherapist

Following a cancer diagnosis, things usually get rolling quickly regarding cancer treatment protocols. However, the patient's emotional needs often go unaddressed. Getting Off the Emotional Roller Coaster, is a wonderful resource filled with practical tools and suggestions for patients, doctors and other caregivers that will help enable the cancer patient to achieve and maintain emotional wellness not only during treatment, but beyond into survivorship as well.

Nancy Stordahl, Cancer Survivor and Author

As a Breast Cancer Nurse Navigator, (seeing an average of 375 newly diagnosed breast cancers a year), and a breast cancer survivor, the treatment and surgery are only a fraction in the equation of the road to recovery. Dr. Barr is so on track with the extreme importance of emotional healing being equally as important as the treatment itself. Her book is tremendous!

Dana McGuirk, Breast Cancer Navigator

GETTING OFF THE EMOTIONAL ROLLER COASTER OF CANCER

A Toolbox for Patients, Survivors, Family Members & Caregivers

Niki Barr, Ph.D.

GETTING OFF THE EMOTIONAL ROLLER COASTER OF CANCER

© 2014 by Niki Barr, Ph.D.

Published by Anchor Rose Publishing
POB 193
Colleyville, Texas 76034

Visit www.CancerEmotionalWellbeing.com

This book may be purchased in bulk for educational, business, fundraising or sales promotional use. For information, please email Niki@CancerEmotionalWellbeing.com.

ISBN: 978-0-9905859-0-9

Printed in the United States of America

Cover and Interior Design: Deana Riddle

The information contained in this book is distributed on an "as is" basis without warranty. *It does not take the place* of talking with your healthcare provider about your *medical* condition or your treatment. While every precaution has been taken in the preparation of this book, neither the author nor the publisher shall have any liability to any person or entity with respect to loss or damage caused or alleged to be caused directly or indirectly by the instructions contained in this book or by the computer hardware or software products described in it.

Dedication

Cancer leaves its imprint on every patient, survivor, family member and caregiver.

I dedicate this book to every one of you, sending you hope and a lighted candle for moving forward with emotional wellbeing.

Acknowledgements

Much appreciation goes to all of those who said, "Yes! You must write this book!"

To all that have entrusted me to listen and guide them in psychotherapy sessions.

To my husband and children who continually supported me with inspiration and love. To my mother who stayed "put" at the finish line, ever cheering me on. To my best friend, Karen, who "gets me" completely. And to all of my other truly magnificent, handholding friends who never let go.

To my editor Rhonda Fleming and to my book producer Deana Riddle, who answered every question ever asked about writing and completion with tremendous dedication and kindness. And to my friend, Helena Iannaccone, RN, MSN, ANP, AOCNP, for her help with medical terminology.

To my coaches, who provided brilliant guidance: Geoffrey Berwind, Martha Bullen, Jack Canfield, Bill Harrison, and Steve Harrison.

Thank you!

Table of Contents

FOREWORD

"What's that?"

It was 3:00am on May 16, 2012, and I had just rolled out of bed for a short walk to my usual middle-of-the-night tinkle. At the then age of 56, I had long ago given up the idea of ever completely sleeping through the night without at least one bathroom run, and I expected to accomplish my watery objective quickly and return to bed to finish out the night.

What should have only taken a minute, instead changed my life forever. In the bathroom, my hand had just accidentally brushed against my right testicle and I jolted fully awake, perspiration instantly breaking out on my forehead and upper lip. The testicle was the size of a tennis ball.

"What's that?"

Up to this point, perhaps like you, I was in perfect health. Never smoked, only occasionally had wine or a vodka martini (three olives), was trim and exercised moderately. I had (and continue to have) fulfilling work, a wonderful social life and a home in a charming town on the Main Line outside of Philadelphia. All my ducks seemed to have—finally—formed into a very pleasant and productive row.

I've since realized that it's only ducks that get in a row - not we humans - and when I found that unexpected swollen growth, I knew something was suddenly terribly amiss. Within a few hours I was in my doctor's office and, as he examined me, I noted that he maintained a poker face. The first intimation I had that this was the very thing I most feared was after he left the examination room. I was still half-dressed, shivering on the examination table. The doctor had left the door slightly open and from the reception desk I overheard the nurse making a phone call to a urologist on my behalf. I slid closer to the partly opened door in time to hear her whisper into the phone "cancer." My emotional roller coaster began at that moment.

What followed is probably quite familiar to you. I met with the urologist, quickly had surgery to remove the inflamed gland, waited far too long for the biopsy report, received the phone call that it was malignant but had not spread, met with oncologists to determine whether to a) do nothing further, b) receive chemotherapy, or c) undergo a "short course" of targeted radiation treatments.

All of this while still living my life, going to work, being functional and in control, as far as the outside world could judge. My close friends gathered round and I felt supported both logistically and emotionally during this initial period.

As the weeks unfolded, though, I observed firsthand that people hate the C-word. Your closest relationships want to support you, but I also realized, from subtle cues, that they want you to "get through it" and in reality don't want to talk about it too much. You want to talk about it a lot in order to process your emotions. They will listen to you, but they're scared, too, and want everything to return to normal as quickly as possible. I mean, we're Americans, right? Get on with it! You're fine! Be strong!

In the months that followed my radiation treatments, I experienced unpredictable energy collapses due to my white blood count being affected by the radiation. These compounded the anxiety I had been living with anyway, but they eventually subsided and I got my energy back. Outwardly, everything had returned to normal.

But nothing was as before and nothing was "normal." Once things stabilized, my dear ones, who had faithfully supported me, felt they could put it all behind them. But for me, there was nothing to "put behind." While I was in crisis mode through the surgery, diagnosis and treatments, it was easy to stay focused on what I needed to do for my body. But when that all passed and my body began to heal, then the emotional backlash hit me. I had gone through what had long been my primal fear: getting a dread disease. I was now a cancer survivor (I hate that term...).

Over the next eighteen months, filled with follow-up MRI's and X-rays, I experienced the emotional roller coaster Niki deals with in this book. I found myself in a new world where no one really wanted to be reminded that cancer had hit me. I became downcast and the ever-present and unexpressed anxiety made me moody. It was a lonely part of my cancer journey. I eventually learned from other cancer fighters that this is common and, thankfully, I was able to come out the other side of this and am a stronger person for it. Niki's advice has played a major role on my path to emotional healing.

I invite you to read what follows with an open and optimistic heart. Niki has taught me to regard my body - and my emotions - not as the enemy who gave me cancer, but as the "friend" who all along has been trying to cure and comfort me during this challenge. She has made a world of difference to my emotional health, my state of mind, and my hopes. And she'll do the same for you.

Onwards!

Geoffrey Berwind, Cancer Fighter - 2012-present
www.StorytellingSuccess.com

INTRODUCTION

Getting Off the Emotional Roller Coaster of Cancer was written for each of you—cancer patient, cancer survivor, family member and caregiver. It was written because the emotional shock of cancer and the emotions of cancer are glaringly in your face, and no one, to any great extent, acknowledges them or helps you know what to do with them. And when emotions are ignored, like a volcano, they will either spew or erupt—neither of which is helpful for emotional wellbeing or physical healing.

As a psychotherapist who has seen thousands of people dealing with cancer over the years, I've heard things like:

> Cancer came out of nowhere. I'm a healthy person and I got smacked with a diagnosis. Why?

> I'm cancer free! Yay!! After the celebration, everyone expects me to just go back to being the same person I was. But I'm not the same person I was and I never will be. Cancer changed me.

> I don't know what I'm supposed to say to her. She looks awful and feels awful. She wants to talk to me about it, but I don't want to hear it. I'm terrified of cancer. I know I'd just start bawling if we talked about it. It takes everything I have to keep "it" down when I see her.

> I'm exhausted. They say I need to take time for myself, but how am I supposed to do that? I'm running him to the doctor, cooking for him and then he doesn't want to eat it, picking up prescriptions, trying to keep up with the insurance and everything else. I love him. I just don't know how much longer I can do this.

Cancer forces change. No one touched by cancer is ever exactly the same as he/she was before cancer. How could you be?

Getting Off the Emotional Rollercoaster of Cancer is focused on giving you numerous tools for coping with your thoughts and emotions within cancer. I divided the book into sections so you can read specifically what pertains to you at a particular time.

These sections include:

> Diagnosis
>
> Medical Treatment
>
> Surviving Cancer
>
> Metastasis, Recurrence and Late Effects
>
> Grief, Death and Loss
>
> Emotional Wellness, Empowered Living
>
> Resources

The first five sections focus on specific parts of the cancer journey.

Next you'll find a section entitled Emotional Wellness and Empowered Living. The purpose of this section is to help you explore and examine yourself from a deeper, more insightful place. It incorporates your core self, your spiritual, physical, and emotional self, and is focused on living from empowerment—instead of feeling powerless.

The final section of the book is titled Resources. At the very beginning of this section is a list of the emotions covered in the book and the section where you can find the tools for dealing with that particular emotion. Regardless of where you are within cancer, you can turn to this section and quick-ly find tools to address whatever emotion you need help with at the moment.

Next you will find sources of additional reading, CD's, organi-zations, and other materials you may find helpful.

I wrote this book because I believe emotional wellbeing is extremely important to your healing process. While cancer strikes all ages and has many forms—sometimes involving death—it always evokes emotions.

You must be able to feel what you feel, express what you feel, and have tools to cope with your thoughts and feelings. Then you'll be able to get off the cancer emotional roller coaster, even if only for five minutes at a time.

That is the goal of this book.

SECTION 1

THE EMOTIONAL SHOCK OF CANCER DIAGNOSIS

"Within us all there are wells of thought and dynamos of energy which are not suspected until emergencies arise."

Thomas J. Watson, Sr.

YOUR EMOTIONS

Sheer terror is not an uncommon response to the words "you have cancer." After hearing that news, your mind automatically shuts down to protect itself—making it virtually impossible to hear anything else your doctor tells you.

Susan returned to her doctor for the results of a breast biopsy, expecting a good report. The biopsy had been ordered as a precaution, since her doctor believed all was well. But it wasn't. Susan had breast cancer. All she could think about was getting out of that office as fast as possible. But instead she sat frozen to her chair.

Jim went to the doctor for tests, complaining of how tired he was and that he had noticed his neck was swollen on one

1

side, just under his jaw. When the doctor told him his test results indicated Stage IV head and neck cancer, a rush of tears began streaming down his face. He could hear the doctor asking him questions, but no answers would come. Jim wondered if he was having a nightmare because nothing was making sense in that moment.

Ryan's wife, a labor and delivery nurse, was worried that something was terribly wrong with her husband. He had a cough that wouldn't go away, despite over the counter medicine and two rounds of antibiotics. But then, he didn't cough all the time, just some times. And it was allergy season. Finally, she convinced him to go to the doctor. The doctor ordered a chest X-ray followed by scans and biopsy and Ryan was called to come in for an appointment to discuss the results—Stage III lung cancer. Ryan was stunned. He angrily told the doctor it had to be a mistake because he didn't smoke.

Story after story shows how a cancer diagnosis slams the patient and family members alike—whether or not they were expecting to hear those words: "You have cancer." Emotional shock takes over, often intertwined with disbelief and denial, and this is a normal response.

Coping With the Words "You Have Cancer"

How do you cope with a cancer diagnosis? Well, at first you DON'T. You let yourself feel what you feel.

> You cry.
>
> You scream.
>
> You run.
>
> You go numb.

You panic.

You write about it.

You talk about it.

You pray.

You cradle your dog or your cat.

You surround yourself with family.

You call your best friend.

You want time alone.

Usually alarms are going off, telling you to do something. Take action. Fix this. But it's better to give yourself time to emotionally react to the news. If you can, take a few days, a week, or whatever time possible to sift and sort through your thoughts and feelings before you jump into considering treatment options.

FAMILY EMOTIONS

When you learn your loved one has a cancer diagnosis, whether you are with them at the doctor's office or you find out later, you too can experience tremendous emotional shock. In my professional experience, family members are faced with a double whammy. Not only do you have to cope with your loved one's illness, you also have to cope with your own emotions. Sometimes family members have a more difficult time dealing with the diagnosis than the cancer patient. Therefore, you must take time for yourself, to "take in" your loved one's cancer diagnosis.

When Judy came home from work, she was alarmed to see her husband's car already in the garage. She always got home first and had dinner ready when John arrived, typically an hour later. But today when she walked in the door and saw John sitting on the couch with his head in his hands, she knew something was horribly wrong.

Without thinking, Judy ran to him asking, "What's going on?" John answered in a broken whisper, "I have prostate cancer." Judy forced herself to stay calm, even though she wanted to scream at the top of her lungs, "WHY?" John was the kindest man she knew, always stopping to help others. And besides, he took excellent care of his body, always eating well and exercising regularly. Judy choked back tears and tremendous anger. Nothing could have prepared her for this. She didn't even know John had a doctor's appointment.

Kristen had driven her partner Tracey to the emergency room because she was in a lot of pain. The pain was coming from her right side, around her stomach. Kristen was certain Tracey had appendicitis and expected emergency surgery to be ordered. Emergency surgery was ordered, and the doctor found a large tumor which was diagnosed as appendiceal cancer. Tracey was shaken. But Kristen began having chest pains which were diagnosed as a full-blown panic attack.

Emotional shock is a normal response to your loved one's cancer diagnosis. Give yourself time to emotionally digest what's happening with your loved one. While you want to do something *right now* to help—like immediately getting a second opinion, arguing with test results, or having a family meeting to let everyone know—your emotions should be addressed first. Give yourself a 'time out' as soon as you can.

Talk with a good friend.

Go out in nature and run/walk/sit.

Call your friend who is in the medical field.

Rest.

Meditate.

Listen to music.

Pray.

Write.

Paint.

Clean.

Swim.

Feel what you feel.

Emotions stemming from a cancer diagnosis—whether you are the patient, a family member, or a friend—are normal and can swing from rage to panic to deep sadness, or any other number of feelings. Emotions accompany emotional shock.

EMOTIONAL WELLNESS FOR ALL

Understanding What Emotions Are

Emotions are quite simply like little children. They don't "get" logic. You can feel scared and try to ease your 'scaredness' by spending time thinking through what is happening, writing down positive affirmations, or reading an article on how to get through your fear. But you're still scared. You might try to convince yourself everything will be fine, but you still feel scared. You simply can't explain away an emotion.

Many people try very hard *not* to feel what they're feeling. They often try to push emotions down, but in the end they will come back up. Think volcano! Emotions that have been pushed down will eventually erupt. And in my experience as a psychotherapist, they come up and out with even more intensity. While we aren't taught to allow emotions to be expressed, they are normal. And that doesn't get said enough. You need to feel what you feel–especially with a cancer diagnosis.

Emotions are Unpredictable

Sara was walking down the aisle at the grocery store she has shopped at for many years. She actually likes shopping at this particular store because nothing ever changes. The ketchup is always where the ketchup is and the toilet paper is always were the toilet paper is. Sara finds shopping for groceries relaxing, since all that's required of her is to go down the aisles putting items in the cart.

But today is different. Sara notices tears are flying down her face, even though she wasn't even thinking about her father's cancer diagnosis. As a matter of fact, she came to the grocery store so she didn't have to think. And now a stranger is asking if she is okay and offering her a Kleenex.

Emotions are like that. Sometimes they show up when you least expect them. Tim was with a customer who was asking numerous questions about a particular product. Tim had sold computer software for years and, being very familiar with it, easily answered the customer's questions. But then Tim found himself getting angry and impatient—wanting the customer to either buy it or not. Tim was hugely surprised, since he prided himself on his patience. After the conversation ended, Tim stared into space trying to make sense of it. Immediately he thought about the scheduled doctor's visit coming up later in the week to discuss his cancer treatment options.

You really can't know when, where, or how your emotions

will present themselves. They are similar to a cloudless sky suddenly filling with storm clouds that seem to come out of nowhere.

Asking "Why Me?"

I've heard many people say that they didn't ask "why me" when they got a cancer diagnosis. And I've heard just as many people say they did. Whether cancer runs in the your family or not, it's perfectly normal to wonder, "Why me?"

As human beings we naturally want to make sense of our experience.

I'm a good person. Why me?

I eat organic food and exercise every day. Why me?

I get regular medical checkups. Why me?

I'm not fat. Why me?

I go to church, I believe in God, I pray. Why me?

I'd give someone the shirt off my back. Why me?

I've never smoked or taken drugs, Why me?

I don't drink. Why me?

Cancer doesn't run in my family. Why me?

I'm careful to wash off my fruits and vegetables. Why me?

I've been healthy all of my life. Why me?

Many explanations can be found for cancer including genetics, pollution, and chemicals in our environment and food. And I'm sure we could identify other reasons. But when you're looking at a cancer diagnosis for you or your loved one, knowing why will never be enough to take away what now looms in front of you. But still, wondering is normal.

Playing the Blame Game

Why didn't I exercise?

Why did I eat hot dogs, drink soda, eat sugar... and lots of it?

Why didn't she go to the doctor sooner?

Why did I keep working there, inhaling and working with those chemicals every day?

Why didn't he take better care of himself?
Why did I keep smoking?

Why did I take drugs to sleep?

Why didn't he tell me he knew something was wrong with his body?

Why X? (You fill in the blank.)

Blaming yourself or your loved one for getting cancer throws you into an abyss—a black hole. You may feel guilt, shame, and remorse, "beating yourself up" emotionally. But no amount of this pummeling will change the diagnosis.

Instead, try these thoughts and statements:

> *I'll take good care of myself/my loved one through this healing process.*

> *I choose not to blame myself/my loved one for cancer.*

> *I choose to be patient with myself/my loved one.*

Using the word "choose" empowers you. Choosing is an active word, inherently requiring action. On the other hand, blaming yourself feels bad and keeps you "locked" in a cycle of emotional sabotage. Instead of blaming, try this sentence

"I choose to_____."

How does that feel?

Can you feel the difference between blaming and choosing?

Feeling Out Of Control

"Cancer is a term used for diseases in which abnormal cells divide without control and are able to invade other tissues," as defined by the National Cancer Institute. Similarly, *you* may feel "out of control" or that all you can do is go through medical treatment, which is being done *to you*. But, in fact, you *can* take many other actions which help you feel more in control of what's happening to your body and emotions. Tangible behaviors enhance emotional wellbeing. Or more simply, taking specific action feels better than not taking action.

Here are some examples of some specific actions you can take:

> *I will inform myself as much as possible so I can know what to expect and how best to proceed within medical care.*

> *I'll talk with the navigator at the treatment center to familiarize myself with available resources such as massage, psychotherapy, and acupuncture. Research indicates navigators are very helpful following diagnosis.*

> *I'll seek out an oncology-trained therapist to learn strategies for getting through cancer, if I believe this to be helpful.*

> *I'll ask about a support group for me to learn from others how they are navigating cancer, if I think this could be useful.*

> *I'll go on the web or call the national organization for whatever type cancer I have to learn more.*

> *I'll contact community resources that offer assistance.*

These are specific tangible things you can do to help yourself move forward. Focus on tangible actions you can take to help yourself and/or your loved one.

Creating an Emotional Wellbeing Toolbox

Another very useful and tangible activity is to create an emotional wellbeing toolbox. The purpose of the toolbox is to be a place to keep tools you can use and materials you'll need to refer to during and after cancer treatment. Keeping the portable toolbox continually organized and easily accessible will go a long way in decreasing the stress of trying to find needed items that can get scattered.

If you don't already have a suitable container and would rather not spend valuable time shopping for one, there are some available on my website at www.canceremotionalwell-being.com.

Choose a container you like that is the right size to hold:

> Binder with tabs
>
> File folders
>
> Spiral Notebook
>
> Note cards
> Pens and colored markers
>
> This book
>
> A journal

Treasured items like your favorite inspiring quotes, the little red heart your granddaughter gave you, the beautiful shell you found on the beach last year, etc.

You may find it helpful to put together your emotional well-being toolbox with a family member or friend. Decorating it with your favorite colors and with your written affirmations glued to it can bring encouragement every time you see it.

Use the toolbox for:

> Your treasured things that help you move forward emotionally such as poems, religious or spiritual ma-

terial, pictures, CD's, etc.

All of your papers from the doctor in file folders or filed behind tabs in the binder.

An up-to-date list of current medications

Insurance receipts

Printed information about cancer

Community, state, and national resources such as information on support groups

Anything else that would be useful for you

Diagnosis Conversation with Family and Friends

Another emotional shock presents itself as you tell your family and friends about the cancer diagnosis. The news is still new for you and now you're choosing to tell others about it. Expect those you tell to be emotionally shocked. Trying to continue making sense of a diagnosis while watching those you love hear about it can be grueling, sapping much emotional energy.

Before you tell your family and friends, consider:

Who you will tell?

When you will tell them?

How you will tell them?

What you will tell them—all of the information you have or pieces of information?

Do you want another family member to tell them?

Do you want everyone to be together or do you want to tell them individually?

Do you want to ask any to come to the doctor with you, so they can ask their medical questions you don't have the answers to?

Do you want to set up a family meeting with a psycho-therapist?

Other things you've thought of?

Answering these questions in advance can be helpful for making your way through the cancer diagnosis conversation. Nothing can truly smooth the way, but thinking it through can at least help you feel clearer about how to go about it.

ANXIETY: TOOLS FOR COPING

Anxiety is clearly an emotion that runs through all phases of cancer. However, anxiety begins with the diagnosis "you have cancer." Please refer to this chapter as often as needed to gather specific tools to meet anxiety head on.

Definition of Anxiety and Tools

On their website, The University of Maryland Medical Center defines anxiety as "a feeling of fear, dread, and uneasiness." In my work with cancer patients, I define anxiety as an "over the top" connection to life, a powerful energy often stemming from fearful thoughts, ever growing exponentially.

Anxiety clearly affects both cancer patients and their families.

According to the National Institute of Cancer, various aspects of the cancer journey are impacted by the ability to cope with anxiety, such as keeping appointments, treatment and fear of recurrence. Additionally the Institute notes on its website that anxiety may "increase ... pain, affect sleep, and cause nausea and vomiting."

Feeling anxious is very normal and is an emotionally healthy response to cancer. How could you not feel anxious? The key is managing anxiety so it doesn't get out of hand.

LIST OF TOOLS TO COPE WITH ANXIETY

TRIANGLE BREATHING
Simple technique for immediate relief.

'CATCHING' ANXIOUS THOUGHTS
Stop the cycle of anxiety before it accelerates.

MEDITATION
Learn to meditate and practice at least once a day.

LIST FIVE THINGS YOU CAN DO
Keep index cards with you and on them list five things you CAN do.

ASK YOURSELF RIGHT NOW
Ask yourself two easy questions and stop anxiety in its tracks.

'WHAT IF' THINKING
Erase all your "what if" self-talk completely.

FOCUS ON MAKING CHOICES
I am choosing to....

HOW TO BRING CALM BACK TO YOURSELF
A question you want to ask yourself to soothe anxiety.

USING DISTRACTION
Specific tools for distracting yourself.

GROUNDING YOURSELF
A simple strategy for eliminating anxiety *right now*!

MOVING YOURSELF FROM, "I CAN'T HANDLE THIS!"
To "I CAN HANDLE THIS!"

ZOOM IN, ZOOM OUT
How to shift your focus from *anxiety* to a better feeling emotion.

YOUR FAVORITE MOVIE STAR
How she/he can help you with anxiety.

HOW LONG CAN YOU 'BLANK' YOUR MIND
A game you can play for easing anxiety.

LET IT GO AND SHRED IT
A tool you can use this minute for anxiety relief.

JOURNAL
Writing thoughts and feelings on paper.

REFUSE TO LISTEN TO CANCER 'HORROR STORIES'
These only increase anxiety.

'R E L A X' EXERCISE
How to calm yourself quickly by focusing on your breathing.

CHOOSING ONE
'Problem solving' anxiety.

DO THE OPPOSITE OF ANXIETY
Focusing on laughter.

MAKE AN APPOINTMENT WITH A THERAPIST
Particularly one who is oncology-trained. Very helpful!

SUPPORT GROUPS
Try one or two groups to find support for relieving anxiety.

FOCUS ON GOOD NUTRITION
Follow nutritional advice from doctor, nurse, dietician.

FOCUS ON PHYSICAL ACTIVITY
Include daily exercise your doctor has approved.

FOCUS ON RESTORATIVE SLEEP
Tools for enhancing your sleep.

Explanation of Tools to Use for Soothing Anxiety

TRIANGLE BREATHING

Draw a triangle on a piece of paper. On the outer left side of the triangle, in the center of the line, write the letter I. On the outer right side of the triangle, in the center of the line, write the letter E. On the outer edge of the bottom, in the center of the line, write the letter P. I is for Inhale, E is for Exhale, and P is for Pause.

Take a deep breath saying the word "inhale" silently. Breathe in slowly, **I N H A L E.** Then exhale slowly, saying **E X H A L E** silently as you breathe out. After you've exhaled, say the word **P A U S E** silently. In the pause, nothing is going on. You are not inhaling and you are not exhaling. You are simply pausing. When pausing, work with thinking **P A U S E 1, 2, 3, 4.** If the pause feels too long, adjust the numbers until it feels comfortable.

Once you've tried the exercise several times, you can substitute a favorite word, phrase, or color for the word "pause" and for the counted numbers. For example, inhale slowly, exhale slowly, then say **PEACE or CALM or BLUE.** Drag these words out to a count of 4 to get your full pause, or whatever amount of time is comfortable. Using this tool, choose whatever meaningful word, color, or phrase that will enhance relaxation, saying it silently and in a very soothing tone to yourself.

You will want to work with this tool before you need it, since this skill requires practice to be the most effective.

'CATCHING' ANXIOUS THOUGHTS

Many troublesome thoughts, especially anxious ones, are thought over and over again, resulting in feeling anxious. The trick to dealing with anxiety is to "catch" anxious feelings before they intensify. You want to slow down and think through what you are telling yourself about the situation at hand.

Write your thoughts down on a note card, one thought per card. See if you can identify what ONE thought started the chain reaction that resulted in your feeling anxious. Then, identify the second thought coming after the first thought. Continue in this manner, thought after thought, in order.

Now, start with the initial thought leading to your feeling anxious and write down a new thought which doesn't result in feeling anxious. What new thought could you substitute for the first old anxious thought? The new thought is confident and empowering. Continue down the line of thoughts until you have replaced all of them.

MEDITATION

Many CD's are available to help you learn how to meditate or to provide guided imagery for meditation.

Here are two I have created:

Meditation For Relaxation, Niki Barr, PhD
Meditation For Soothing Anxiety, Niki Barr, PhD

Or you can try:

How to Meditate with Pema Chodron: A Practical Guide to Making Friends With Your Mind.
Or

Meditation for Beginners by Jack Kornfield

Or

Guided Mindfulness Meditation by Jon Kabat-Zin

Please see RESOURCES at the back of the book for more meditation tools.

TWO QUESTIONS TO FREQUENTLY ASK YOURSELF

Is this thought helping me or hurting me?

Is this thought moving me forward or moving me backward?

"WHAT IF" THINKING

Refuse to play the "what if" game. What if the cancer has spread? What if medical treatment doesn't work? What if I can't take care of her?

One "what if" question leads to another and then another, often spiraling you into increased anxiety. Awareness is key. Stop yourself immediately when you start asking "what if." Instead, ask yourself the two questions listed in the tool above.

BRINGING "CALM" BACK

Soothe yourself. What would feel especially good right now? A cup of tea, another pillow, listening to some music?

FOCUS ON MAKING CHOICES

"I am choosing to....." Choosing is active and empowering. Make a conscious decision to substitute "I am choosing to" for "I have to", "I don't want to", or "I must."

USING DISTRACTION

Work with this tool BEFORE you need it. Choose a favorite place—at the beach, in the library, taking a drive in the country, etc. Think of everything you can about this scene including colors, smells, people involved, sounds, tastes, and how you feel when you're there. Build it up very clearly in your mind, going over and over it, so when you want to use the "distraction" tool you can quickly recall the place and all the tiny details about it. You might want to come up with two or three of these scenarios.

Use this when you're waiting for a medical procedure, getting a medical procedure, waiting for the one you love to get a medical procedure, or whenever else it would be useful for you.

GROUNDING YOURSELF

Stop anxious thoughts in their tracks by "grounding" yourself or focusing on details. Look closely at the room you are in right now. What color is the carpet, the wall? What pictures are hanging on the walls? What color is the table, the chairs? What do the light fixtures look like? Is there dust on them? How about the person talking to you, what color are her/his eyes? Her/his hair? What is she/he wearing? Being very focused on another set of thoughts interrupts the anxious thoughts you were thinking.

MOVING YOURSELF FROM "I CAN'T HANDLE THIS!"

Yes, you can handle whatever is going on five minutes at a time. You can do anything five minutes at a time. Remind yourself you CAN get through the next five minutes and the next five minutes after that. Soon you will look back and notice you've gotten through a bunch of five-minute time blocks.

ZOOM IN, ZOOM OUT

Think of a camera. You can zoom in for a close-up or you can take a regular picture. Using the same idea, you can check in with yourself to see how things are going by zooming in. Ask yourself, "How am I feeling? How are things going in my world? How am I in my immediate surroundings?" Then zoom out and ask, "How am I in the 'big picture' in relation to family members and friends? My community? Life in general?" Using Zoom In/Zoom Out gives you a quick reading of how things are going from a balanced perspective. Are there any adjustments needed to be made up close? How about in the big picture?

Zooming out, in particular, provides relief from anxiety. Since anxiety tends to be focused on what's in your immediate "up close" attention, choosing to pull back (zoom out) brings perspective and balance. For example, "I'm not the only one who has gone through this." "I wonder if I could find resources in places I haven't even thought of," leading you into problem solving and away from various degrees of anxiety.

YOUR FAVORITE MOVIE STAR

Choose a movie star you admire, one who is calm and confident. Imagine how that movie star would handle the situation you are in. What would she/he say to the doctor, to the friend who is offering endless advice, to the insurance company? You've heard the saying "fake it 'til you make it." Put on *your* "calm and confident" to help manage anxiety.

HOW LONG CAN YOU BLANK YOUR MIND?

See how long you can blank your mind, not thinking any thought. Can you do it for five seconds? Ten seconds? Longer? Sometimes it's helpful to let your mind rest. Cancer brings an abundance of things to deal with medically, emotionally, within relationships, etc. Taking a "thought break" can bring much needed respite, if only for a few seconds at a time. You'll find the more you use this tool, the greater amount of time you'll be able to sustain the "thought break."

LET IT GO AND SHRED IT

In her book *The Artist's Way*, Julia Cameron discusses the morning pages exercise—writing three pages of thoughts and feelings each morning before you do anything else. This is an excellent tool for "dumping out" thoughts and feelings.

Many people I've worked with were very hesitant to use this tool because they were concerned someone would find and read what they wrote. To alleviate this concern, I suggested shredding their pages after completing them. The tool became even more powerful when focusing on "letting go" of troublesome thoughts and feelings as the papers were being shredded.

JOURNAL

Journaling, on the other hand, is a progression of thoughts and feelings you write down as desired. Some people find re-reading what they have written very helpful.

A related tool is the video journal. If you have a newer model computer, the camera is built in. You can film yourself discussing thoughts and feelings.

REFUSE TO LISTEN TO CANCER "HORROR" STORIES

Stop listening to cancer "horror stories." Everyone has them and everyone seems ready to tell them without thinking how these stories might affect the listener. When someone starts telling you one, let them know you prefer not to hear those type stories. Then change the subject.

R E L A X EXERCISE

Find a quiet place without distractions. After taking a few slow breaths, inhale while saying "R." Then, exhale while saying "E." Continue in this way spelling the word "RELAX," one letter for each inhale, and one letter for each exhale.

CHOOSING ONE

Make a list of your concerns. Choose one of them and write it down on a note card. What one thing, and ONLY one thing, could you DO to ease your concern? Then do it.

DO THE OPPOSITE OF ANXIETY

What's funny for you? What makes you laugh? Get a joke book, spend time with a friend who "cracks you up," watch a movie that makes you giggle, recall a memory where you laugh every time you think about it.

MAKE AN APPOINTMENT WITH A THERAPIST

This is a tremendous gift you can give yourself, to make an

appointment with a therapist—particularly one who has on-cology training. Together the two of you will navigate cancer, moving forward, focused on emotional wellbeing.

SUPPORT GROUPS

Support groups can be wonderful for providing both infor-mation and emotional support. Some people hesitate to go to these. But I recommend you at least check several out to see how a group could benefit you.

FOCUS ON GOOD NUTRITION

Eat well, consulting your doctor about what foods will be best. Some treatment centers or resource centers have dieti-cians who will provide important information for your diet within cancer.

FOCUS ON PHYSICAL ACTIVITY

After discussing physical activity with your doctor, do what-ever is permissible. Do what you can do. Studies continually indicate people feel better both physically and emotionally when exercise is part of their daily routine.

FOCUS ON RESTORATIVE SLEEP

There are many CD's or MP3 downloads on the market that help with sleep.
Try:

Sleep Through Insomnia by KRS Edstrom

Or

Just Relax- Relaxing to Sleep CD, by Gail Seymour

Please see RESOURCES at the back of this book for more restorative sleep tools.

DEEP HEALING RESOURCES

The above suggestions are very practical and extremely effective when dealing with the anxiety brought on by a cancer diagnosis. In addition, I have included an entire section in this book (Section 6) for anyone interested in learning about deep emotional healing. This type of healing deals with your emotional health at a much deeper level. The exercises are more intangible and require a greater investment of time, energy, and emotion, but the results last longer and are more comprehensive, affecting every area of your life in a positive way.

SUMMARY

The emotional shock that comes with hearing "you have cancer" is both unnerving and frightening. Typical emotions within diagnosis include anger, sadness, hopelessness, overwhelm, confusion, numbness and anxiety. Taking time for assimilating your feelings in response to a diagnosis is essential before diving into treatment options. Feeling what you feel and understanding why you must feel what you feel is a powerful component for moving forward.

Creating an emotional wellbeing toolbox is a tangible activity that, whether undertaken alone or with someone you love, is useful for moving into treatment and beyond. It holds both tools for your own wellbeing and the myriad of papers and information you will be receiving throughout cancer.

While many emotions are common in pre-treatment, anxiety is especially dominant. This section provided many tools for meeting anxiety head-on—tools designed to help you cope and manage this emotion.

In the next session, we'll explore medical treatment. You will want to gather as much accurate information as possible about the cancer and treatment options, once you've given yourself time for "absorbing" news of the diagnosis. Within treatment, emotional wellbeing is essential in order for you and your family to move forward through cancer.

Sources for This Section Include:

http://annonc.oxfordjournals.org/content/23/suppl_10/x302.full

http://crd.sagepub.com/content/9/1/39.refs

http://jco.ascopubs.org/content/32/1/3.full

http://www.umgcc.org/patient_info/index.htm

http://www.cancer.gov/cancertopics/pdq/supportivecare/adjustment/patient

Julia Cameron, The Artist's Way (New York: Penguin Putnam Inc., 2002).

SECTION 2

THE EMOTIONAL SHOCK OF MEDICAL TREATMENT

The only courage that matters is the kind that gets you from one moment to the next.

Mignon McLaughlin

YOUR EMOTIONS

Now that you've taken time to "absorb" the news of your diagnosis and have gathered all the information you can about your type of cancer and the treatment options available, it's time to make a decision about your treatment and move forward.

Surgery, radiation and chemotherapy are powerful enemies of cancer and are used separately, together, or in some combination for healing and eradicating cancer. But no matter which treatment option(s) you choose, emotions will definitely accompany the treatment. And this chapter will help you be prepared for them and give you some tools to deal with them.

Justin never questioned his ability to deal with whatever happened in his life. Colleagues and even his boss talked with Justin about what they should do when facing difficult situations. Family and friends consistently asked Justin for help solving challenging problems.

So Justin wasn't worried at all when his doctor advised him to have surgery followed by chemo to address Stage II colon cancer. Justin went in for surgery and recovered fairly easily, despite an infection. Justin attended chemo education, learning all about what would be involved. Again, Justin was fine and even looked forward to chemo so he could get on with his life.

But on the first day of chemo, sitting in that chair with nurses and patients all over the room, a nurse moved toward him to get the infusion started. Justin looked at a woman sitting next to him with a shaved head and suddenly fierce anxiety sparked. Justin heard himself saying to the nurse, "I can't do this!"

Here are some statements from a breast cancer patient:
"You're saying you want to radiate where I had breasts?"
"But there must be another way, surely a green drink or meditation...the cancer isn't findable anymore,...this is just wrong."
"I need to be getting married right now and thinking about having children."

Carol had taken so many doses of chemo she'd lost track. Her doctor had recommended one after another in hopes something would help her, but nothing did. He suggested she be part of a clinical trial she was eligible for. But Carol had had enough treatment. Feeling hopeless and depressed, she decided to take a break from treatment.

It's normal to think:

"You're doing what to my body?" "Seriously?"

And responding:

"NO! I absolutely DO NOT want to do this,"

BUT you get treatment anyway. You do so because your doctor recommends you do and because these are considered to be the best medical bombs we have in our arsenal right now to blast out, shrink, and heal cancer.

On the other hand, some people choose complementary and alternative medicines. According to the National Center for Complementary and Alternative Medicine's website, complementary medicine is typically
used with conventional medicine whereas alternative medicine is used instead of conventional medicine. This group of health approaches includes: tai chi, meditation, biofeedback, herbs, supplements, acupuncture, etc.

Regardless of the treatment option(s) you choose to follow, traditional medical treatment packs yet another emotional shock. No longer are you conversing about a cancer diagnosis, you are now doing something about the cancer. Tangible does feel better, but still emotions are affected and are typically a roller coaster ride consisting of confusion, fear, worry, hopelessness, feeling overwhelmed, etc.

FAMILY EMOTIONS

Family members' emotions, without a doubt, are enormous to deal with. You're caught up thinking about your loved one, often worried about cancer treatment options, providing emotional support, and dealing with your own emotions. You, too, deal with emotional shock.

Kara and her partner Chris went together to see the doctor for treatment options concerning Chris's ovarian cancer. They had spent the weekend trying to make sense of it all. Chris had simply gone in for gallbladder surgery when the cancer was found. Having cancer never crossed their mind, but now it was a mind-blowing reality.

Kara didn't want Chris to know how worried she was. What would happen to their life together? Would Kara be able to support both of them financially? And what if Chris needed Kara to be her caregiver? Then what?

Endless questions rocked her mind while she tried to stay as calm as possible when talking with Chris.

Nick was certain his brother would come through head and neck cancer just fine. He had done quite a lot of research and was pleased with Jim's
doctor. Nick felt surprised each time Jim began to say things like, "Maybe I won't make it," or "I probably won't be able to go on our fishing trips ever again." Nick found himself continually reassuring Jim.

Jason had always been close to his mom. He was the oldest and had needed to help out financially from time to time, since his dad was disabled.

Jason was at the appointment when the doctor told his mom she had terminal lung cancer. The doctor suggested trying an aggressive form of chemotherapy that would not cure, but would possibly add some time to her life. Jason wanted to scream. "Why put my mother through chemo to hopefully bank a few more months of life?" He felt caught between suggesting no treatment and his parents' decision to pursue medical treatment.

Emotional shock weighs in as you try to make sense of what is happening to your loved one and what is happening to you in response to your loved one's circumstances. You may feel angry, wondering if the doctor is compassionate enough and/or doing enough to help your loved one. You may feel helpless, wishing you were going through cancer instead of your loved one. Or you may be in denial, truly believing your loved one does not have cancer at all. You could find yourself feeling all of these at the same time, in different combinations, or a variety of other feelings.

Expect to experience various emotional shocks throughout your loved one's treatment. Just know that this is normal.

EMOTIONAL WELLNESS FOR ALL

Understanding What Emotional Shock Is

For the sake of our conversation regarding treatment, I'm defining emotional shock as hyper-vigilant emotions constantly on guard as a result of changes occurring within treatment. These may be physical changes in your body or tangible treatment changes.

Think about watching the news. When you turn the TV on a news channel, the word "ALERT" is going across the screen at the bottom. The word "alert" immediately gets our attention. We wonder what has happened. Our emotions perk up and stay heightened as we begin to grasp the latest tragedy. Within cancer, because it's happening to you or your loved one's body, each change signals an "alert," often bringing another emotional shock—or hyper-vigilant emotions.

In my psychotherapy experience, emotional shock in treatment is not a one-time event. Instead, you may be dealing with it at the onset of treatment, in the middle, and again when finishing treatment. Or you may get through the initial phases of treatment just fine and later in treatment find yourself dealing with it. Or emotional shock may follow you throughout all of cancer. Emotional shock is unpredictable, yet important to deal with. The key is not getting caught off guard, realizing that it's normal, and having a strategy to deal with it.

Cancer is dynamic. It doesn't necessarily stay in one place or respond to any given treatment. Based on scan results, lab results, etc., treatment is changed to offer optimal outcomes. The change is what stimulates the emotional shock.

I've seen some patients "tough it out," refusing to allow their feelings to surface. And some patients are very perky, very positive, again not voicing what they are authentically feeling or not allowing anyone else to know what's going on with them. But like we discussed in the first section of the book (Cancer Diagnosis), emotions will certainly emerge at some point.

On the other hand, some patients feel overwhelmingly hopeless and helpless, regardless of the treatment. What started as an initial emotional shock with the diagnosis, that perhaps was not dealt with appropriately, persists throughout treatment. And sometimes when an emotional shock isn't acknowledged, an emotional "numbing" unfolds.

Coping With Emotional Shock and Treatment

Knowing emotional shock is normal and being on the lookout for it, allows you more leverage for choosing your response. Exploring treatment options, going through treatment, and processing the changes that may occur, in you and in your relationships, are times for coping with emotional shock.

TREATMENT OPTIONS

Ask Questions

Information calms emotions. Thoroughly understanding your options for treatment, expected treatment outcome, and side effects is a powerful first step.

Write down a list of questions, every question you have. Then discuss these with at least one family member or friend. Get their input. What would your family member or friend want to know?

Make a new list including your questions and whatever you found beneficial to you that your family member or friend contributed.

Schedule an appointment with your doctor to discuss treatment options. Even if these have already been discussed with you upon diagnosis, you can't possibly "hear" them at that time.

Having a list of specific questions empowers you to both learn what your options are and make a decision about treatment. It is just as empowering for your family members to understand your options and what you are considering. Good questions for a loved one to ask may include:

1. How can I best support you regarding medical treatment options?

2. Would you like me to do research with you on treatment options?

3. If so, what would be most helpful for you?

Knowledge is powerful for settling fear, anxiety, depression, and every other emotion. That said, emotions come with cancer, regardless of how much you know. Allow yourself to feel what you feel.

Doctor Appointment

Take a family member or friend with you to the doctor appointment. Having two sets of ears helps sort through what was said after the appointment. Decide before the appointment who will write down the answers.

Ask every single one of the questions on your list. You wrote each one down because it was important to you to know the answers. Do not let yourself leave without them.

Many times I'm told in psychotherapy sessions that people leave a doctor's appointment dissatisfied, reasoning:

> *I didn't want to take up too much time. My doctor is busy.*

> *My questions sounded dumb.*

> *I didn't want to make my doctor mad with all of these questions, especially since he or she will be taking care of me.*

I just didn't want to ask that. It's embarrassing.

I don't want my doctor to think I'm doubting him or her.

My doctor seemed distracted, so I just skipped over some questions.

Does it really matter what I ask? They're going to do whatever needs to be done anyway.

The nurse kept coming in and interrupting. Maybe I can ask these questions later.

I didn't think the doctor knew the answers to my questions. He or she seemed confused.

My doctor asked the medical student what he thought the answer was. I didn't like having a student answer my questions, so I stopped asking.

My doctor just doesn't have a good bedside manner. I should just trust what he or she is going to do.

Get your questions answered satisfactorily for yourself. Of course, there is a lot that is still not known. However, why would you stay with a doctor who doesn't help you understand treatment?

Consider This:

Most likely you've gone into the doctor's office feeling some degree of overwhelm. If you leave without getting your questions answered to your satisfaction, that degree of overwhelm jumps higher. You need to know as much as you can about what will happen to your body.

It is your body. Nobody else will be physically going through what you are—including your family members and friends. While you may be given a great deal of advice about what to choose, you must be the one who decides.

Your doctor doesn't have all of the answers and doesn't know exactly what will happen. He or she can only give you their best opinions.

If you leave the doctor's office dissatisfied that your questions weren't taken seriously or weren't answered with information you could understand, you may want to get a second opinion. Most doctors agree with getting second opinions.

You **must** feel confident about your doctor's knowledge and ability to carry out your chosen treatment option.

Having a compassionate doctor who understands how difficult treatment is for your body and your emotions is both validating and very helpful for moving forward through cancer.

Choosing Treatment

Regardless of what treatment option you choose, even if only one is available, keep the focus on choice. "I'm choosing to" is empowering and soothing for your emotions.

This is not saying you like what will happen to your body. Of course you won't. But, knowing within yourself that you are, in fact, CHOOSING to go with treatment goes a long way to feeling more in control and, therefore, to comforting your anxiety to some degree.

BEGINNING MEDICAL TREATMENT –YOUR EMOTIONS

It is not unusual for the first day of medical treatment to usher in a flood of emotions. Whether you are going in for surgery, getting your port put in for chemo, getting chemo, or going to radiation, your physical and emotional self is forever changed.

Jeanette's best friend Sheila was so upbeat and positive. She had had a double mastectomy followed by chemo and radiation. She continually worked to reassure Jeanette who had just been diagnosed with breast cancer. While Jeanette appreciated her friend's cheerleading, inside she felt completely overwhelmed. Jeanette found herself still trying to cope with her diagnosis. But now, here she was on her way to the operating room to get a double mastectomy.

Kevin figured radiation would be okay. He was way more scared of chemo. While walking from the waiting room to the room for his radiation treatment, he noticed his heart was racing. He was seriously considering re-scheduling for another day. Somehow he managed to talk intelligently to the nurse as she was getting him ready.

Shayla had come in for chemo education, but nothing could prepare her for sitting in the chair next to the woman with the bald head. She knew her head would look the same in a few weeks. Tears rolled down her cheeks as she tried to answer the nurse's questions.

Emotions are often wrapped with such questions as:

How will I ever get through this?

What will happen to me?

Why is that nurse so perky?

Why is everyone acting like this is no big deal?

What if I die right here, right now?

Does anyone have any idea how this is affecting me?

What if I get an infection? I wonder if the doctor/nurse washed their hands?

What if the doctor/nurse screws this up accidently?

How could this be happening right now?

Could I just leave?

FAMILY EMOTIONS

"I can't believe my sweetheart is having a port put in for chemo. She's getting this thing inserted under her skin today. What will happen to her, to us, to our family now and once she starts getting chemo?"

"The navigator assured us we could talk with her as much as we wanted about Diane's treatment. I'm glad for that. What a relief!"

James brought Ben to radiation. He was relieved to sit in the waiting room. He talked a good game...all would be okay... everything was fine...many people got cancer and survived. But privately he was very nervous, even wondering if any of this was really necessary.

You may wonder:

Why is it she's the one going through it and isn't worried at all? Really?

What am I supposed to do? How should I act?

What if I'm doing the wrong thing, saying the wrong thing?

Do they know if this chemo/radiation/surgery is a good thing? I know they said it was, but how certain are they?

What will happen when we go home?

What If I can't handle seeing my loved one go through treatment?

Will our lives ever be the same?

What if I get sick?

Emotions can get confusing and overwhelming as you focus on providing support to your loved one. It's normal not to want to show your true emotions, yet often, doing so brings closeness. Your loved one, in my experience, "feels" your fear, worry, and dread on some level.

EMOTIONAL WELLNESS FOR ALL

In my clinical experience, medical treatment involves the one going through it and everyone in their immediate circle. Medical treatment does not happen in isolation. Therefore, it is essential to pull together and move forward through treatment together. If you can, work with a therapist—individual therapy, couple therapy, and/or family therapy—to help navigate cancer emotions and concerns. Treatment centers are now beginning to offer this service at no charge or with a nominal charge.

Family Meetings

Sometimes family isn't physically or emotionally available or there is no family. If that's true for you, skip to the next section.

Family meetings are essential for keeping everyone informed of what's going on within treatment and for both providing and receiving needed support. There are many ways to set up family meetings. What's most important is structuring these meetings according to what works best for your family.

Suggested Structure for Family Meeting

Schedule a time to meet regularly that fits with everyone's schedule as much as possible. For example, Sunday afternoon at 4 or Thursday evening at 7. The key is to "show up," making a commitment to be there.

Meetings seem to work best when held for one hour and no more than an hour and a half.

If age appropriate, children are welcome to be involved. Or have a separate family meeting so they, too, understand what's happening to their loved one.

Choose one family member to be the moderator of the meeting, to keep things moving along. It is a good idea for notes to be taken and distributed to family.

Family members can submit concerns, questions, and topics ahead of the meeting to the moderator.

Fortunately, many venues are now available for having family meetings. Consider Skype, conference calls, Google+ hangouts, etc., if everyone doesn't live in the same town.

Helpful Family Meeting Rules

Be fully present at these meetings. No TV, texting, computer work, and other distractions. For one hour, dedicate this time to your family.

Only one person speaks at a time, while everyone else listens. This seems basic, yet I've seen family members jump in over each other's words and nothing gets accomplished.

Work with a speaker/listener concept such that: the speaker talks, the listener listens and when the speaker is finished speaking, the listener reflects back what was said. "So you'd like me to keep the calendar of appointments." Then, the listener now becomes the speaker and responds. "I can do that. I will write these on a calendar and let everyone know when scans, doctor appointments, and chemo is happening."

The family meeting is designed to inform and help family members move through treatment together. It is not for arguing and making hurtful comments. If this is happening, agree to end the meeting. Then those involved can sort it out on their own time. Or this may be a good time to schedule a family therapy appointment. Sometimes it is very difficult for family members to stay on course when moving through emotional issues.

The family meeting is not for gossip, drama or pushing one another's "buttons." You know what's sensitive and not helpful. Just don't go there. For this one hour, lay all of that aside, incorporating respect for one another by listening and stating what you have to say kindly.

The priority with family meetings is the person dealing with medical treatment.

> If he or she does NOT want to discuss a particular issue, you don't.

> If he or she does NOT want your input, don't give it.

> If he or she wants to handle treatment differently, your opinion is trumped.

For you who are going through treatment, it is an absolute necessity that these meetings be helpful and supportive for you. At any time you can choose to:

> Ask the topic be changed to a different one.

> Ask for assistance with whatever you're dealing with.

> Ask for emotional support.

> End the meeting if you believe it is not helpful.

If you choose to end the meeting, it would be beneficial to talk with family members about what would help you most, what you need most.

Topics for Conversation Could Include:

> Cancer patient discussing what's going on within treatment, how they're feeling, their progress, what would be most helpful in terms of support.

42

Logistics: who does what, when, where, how.

Concerns with doctor, lab tests, surgery, chemo, radiation, scans, etc.

What a family member has learned about resources such as support groups, community organizations, state organizations, national organizations, etc.

What a family member has learned about clinical research, helpful books, pamphlets, etc.

What went on in a doctor's appointment, with the cancer patient's permission. This includes changes in medication, new treatment regimen, etc.

Your Family Member Becomes a Caregiver

It is not unusual during treatment for a family member or friend to become a caregiver. Sometimes it's all you can do to go through treatment, resting and recovering in between. Energy is not available as it was before cancer for such tasks as working, taking care of the kids, cleaning house, running errands, cooking, etc. Additionally, you may need help with your own needs, such as taking medication, showering, etc.

Some cancer patients get depressed or angry with someone else taking care of them. This is especially difficult if you have previously managed your life independently.

Some family members get depressed or angry at the "need" to take care of their loved one. It's not the person with cancer so much as it's your now needing to step up into a caregiving role, which necessarily requires balancing all of the other things in your life in addition to being a caregiver.

By our definition, another emotional shock now comes for both patient and family member. When you can't take care of yourself as you did before, when you can't take care of life tasks as you did before, emotions spark significantly. It is the same for the family member who is now a caregiver.

Making this transition is often challenging.

Be very gentle with yourself, Patient and Caregiver. You'll want to lean into soothing actions as much as possible. These could include:

> Listen to your favorite music.

> Have a cup of your favorite soup.

> Drink warm tea.

> Journal your thoughts and emotions to release them.

> Talk with your best friend.

> Sit outside and allow nature to distract you.

> Get hugs, give hugs, hug yourself.

Emotional Conflicts Between Patient and Caregiver

Emotional conflicts are normal, as you've both moved into a new arena, Patient and Caregiver. Sometimes, you may experience emotional shock, but your loved one doesn't, or vice versa. When this occurs, emotions can flair, causing an additional layer of distress.

Jo Anne was helping her sister Jane get through breast cancer. Jo Anne believed her sister needed to eat more and was always putting food in front of Jane, telling her she needed to eat to keep up her strength. Jane ate small meals but did not feel much like eating. After a week of constant "nagging" from her sister, Jane lashed out and told Jo Anne to leave her alone. Jo Anne's feelings were hurt and Jane knew it. But right now she was too fed up to try to fix the situation.

Lyn could see her husband was becoming more depressed each day. She suggested seeing a therapist, but her husband would have nothing to do with it. As the days went by, her husband refused to get out of bed, even asking her to cancel his radiation appointments. Lyn had been reading about depression and believed he was clinically depressed. She decided to talk with the doctor about it by phone. Not surprisingly, the doctor wanted him to come in for an appointment, but he refused. Now Lyn found herself tired, emotionally worn out from all of the cheerleading that was going nowhere.

Cory didn't "get" why his wife was so positive all of the time. Did she not understand she had advanced metastatic breast cancer and was probably going to die? He began resenting hearing about the "pink meetings" as he called them. Each time he tried to talk with her about what the doctor said, she always said the same thing, "Why can't you be positive? I'm fine! What's wrong with you?" Their close relationship was quickly falling apart at a time when they both needed to be on the same page.

I encourage you to seek out an oncology-trained therapist or a support group that can help you move through these conflicts. While conflict is normal, being unable to problem solve together fuels an already elevated stress level within the demands of medical treatment.

Your Control—What Happened?

Cancer automatically brings change right smack into the middle of your life. Before cancer, you scheduled your life with kids, work, errands, vacation, etc. While you might have wished for more free time, all in all your life was fairly predictable and followed a weekly plan.

But now, cancer takes center stage. Life revolves around cancer. Why? Because it has to. Your world involves surgery, check-ups, scans, labs, chemo, radiation, doctor appointments, going to the pharmacy, additional doctor appointments with specialists you were referred to.

When you're not doing something medically, you're trying to rest, recover, and catch up on all of the other things that were put aside so you could do what you medically needed to do. Cancer patients, family members, and caregivers often speak of feeling a lack of control of their time. When I ask what that's like emotionally, I hear words like sadness, loneliness, frustration, fear, worry, and overwhelm. Life feels unmanageable.

While cancer is big, really big, you want to begin to focus on what you can control. As we discussed earlier, work with words like:

> *I'm choosing to look at a magazine now.*

> *I will rest now, so I feel better.*

> *No, I've decided not to go to lunch with you today. I'd like to watch a movie at home instead.*

> *I'm just not sleeping well. My doctor's appointment is in three weeks. But I'm not going to wait to talk with her until then. I will call now, so I can move forward with getting this resolved.*

Yes, let's go to dinner. It will feel good to get out of the house for a little while.

Dr. Lane, I'm choosing to eat more of a plant-based diet. I notice I feel better when I do.

I think that nurse practitioner knows a lot and is very good. But she is so busy, I can't get my questions asked and answered. I've asked for an appointment with the other nurse practitioner to see if I feel more comfortable asking her/him my questions.

Each and every time you choose, you assert what's true for you, you bring back "control." Cancer is not about blindly doing whatever everyone tells you to do. Cancer is about taking care of yourself in the process. When you feel more in control of your life, emotional wellbeing is enhanced.

When Treatment Changes Your Appearance

Obviously some medical treatment involves a change to your appearance. A body part is surgically removed, your hair falls out, you "puff out" with fluid, or some other change.

You notice and people notice. Give yourself time to grieve changes in your body. It's okay to cry. It's okay to feel what you feel. When you choose to put this off, you prolong coming to terms with the change. This can lead to self-imposed isolation, feeling bad about yourself, depression, and a host of other self-negating outcomes.

I've worked with many women who choose not to look at themselves in the mirror for a very, very long time after a mastectomy. They no longer see themselves as beautiful or sensuous.

I've worked with men who no longer want to talk about anything with anyone. They feel impatient, frustrated, angry about having a feeding tube.

Women who lose their hair—some hate it and some don't mind it. But those that do hate it feel loss and profound sadness.

Of course people notice, too. Hurtful and often thoughtless comments are made to you or about you, which you happen to overhear. Awkward, frustrating, overwhelming, confusing…you wonder how people can be so insensitive.

In my experience, coming to terms with these changes inside of you through meeting your feelings head-on goes a long way in helping you deal with others' responses and reactions. This doesn't mean they don't hurt or feel pretty awful. But in the end, you are on solid ground, as it were, within yourself.

When Treatment Doesn't Change Your Appearance

When medical treatment doesn't change you appearance, most of the time people won't know you have cancer—unless you or someone else has told them. That can be helpful in and of itself. But sometimes you're having a hard time remembering something due to chemo brain, you may have mouth sores making it difficult to talk, you have neuropathy in your toes and walk very slowly, or something else.

When someone doesn't know what's going on with you or is giving you a hard time, you may want to:

Ignore it.

Tell them flat out "I'm dealing with cancer."

Say, "Yep, side effects of cancer."

Often what happens next is the person wants to know more about your cancer or says to you, "Well you don't look sick." You may want to follow up with:

"Thanks," and change the subject.

Tell them you don't want to discuss cancer.

What Do You Say?

If you can, remember people are very uncomfortable with cancer. Usually they have no clue what to say or what not to say. While many people have cancer in this society, we have not been socialized with what is appropriate to say.

When someone says X, You may want to say Y:

What's happened to you, where is your hair?

I'm healing from chemo, my hair is growing back in.

When people have cancer, sometimes the drugs make your hair fall out.

You have cancer, oh my friend's uncle's cousin had that same kind and he died.

Really? Gosh, I'm taking it a day at a time, so far so good.

Hmmm. Sorry to hear that.

You need to try that green drink with papaya, crushed ants, and skins of grapes in it. My mother's brother's daughter's sister had the same kind of cancer you have and she's just fine.

Well, that's great! Good for her.

Oh, you know, my doctor is taking another route and I'm getting along just fine. Thank you anyway.

Are you going to die?

I don't know.

I don't think so.

Who knows?

You just need to be positive. You can beat this, mind over matter.

We'll see.

That could be true.

Maybe so.

It could be worse. My partner's best friend's aunt's daughter had it way worse than you. You're lucky.

Yes I am.

Yes it could be worse.

Good to know.

How did you get cancer, does it run in your family?

I don't know.

I'm not sure.

God doesn't give you more than you can handle.

Thanks for sharing.

Good to know.

Taking Care of You When Someone Says Something "Dumb"

As previously discussed, people don't really know what's appropriate to say or not to say when cancer is front and center. Take care of yourself by not feeding into the conversation or giving them more to discuss. Disarm their comments by:

Keeping your answers short and to the point.

Tell them, "I don't want to discuss cancer," then change the subject. You may want to lead right into asking a question about how they're doing or feeling. Another option is to ask them a question about their hobby, love interest, kids, etc. People do love to talk about themselves, so choose an enticing topic to ask about.

If a person continues to pursue the topic of cancer, be firm and clear that cancer is off limits for discussion. Sometimes it may be necessary to physically remove yourself, and that's okay, too.

Focus on the idea that it's your body. You can choose to discuss what's going on or you can choose not to. Do not "people please." Do "self please" which leads to self-empowerment and emotional wellbeing.

Body Image, Who I Am Now

Your appearance, your appearance, your appearance. Yes, it does matter to you. And yes, you are ever so grateful you still have your body, no matter how it looks. But still....

You may have experienced physical changes in your body such as:

> Swelling
> Hair loss
> Scars
> Body parts that have been surgically removed
> Weight gain or weight loss
> Sexual changes
> Other changes

Adjusting to who you are now tends to be very difficult for some people. It's yet another emotional shock to process and work through. As we've discussed, allowing yourself to feel what you feel is the foundation of moving forward.

It's important to note I've had quite a few cancer patients tell me in psychotherapy sessions, "I look in the mirror and I don't recognize me any more." "I have no clue who that person is." "I don't look like me and I don't feel like me."

And you are different. You've had medical treatment to help you get through cancer as best as your body can. I think people have a tendency to underestimate the changes that do happen. You weren't told the extent to which you'd change in looks and feelings, because no one really knows exactly what will be involved in medical treatment.

Moving Through Physical and Emotional Shock; Change

Talk with a psychotherapist, social worker, psychologist to help you assimilate changes, grief, loss, etc.

Journal your thoughts and feelings.

Blog your thoughts and feelings.

Check Internet resources. (Look in the Resources section of this book.)

Find a support group that is truly supportive of you.

See what community resources are available.

Talk with a compassionate, trusted friend who listens well.

Talk with your nurse navigator.

Your doctor and medical team work to heal you and they change treatment according to how your body responds. When you first consult with your doctor, you're given a plan for how treatment will take place...but the "kicker" is the unknown. It's impossible to know how your body will respond to a particular treatment until it's underway.

This doesn't change the changes that have already taken place. Sadness, frustration, anger, and overwhelm spew out in psychotherapy sessions with patients saying, "I didn't know this is how I'd look, how I'd feel, what would happen to me." Exactly, because you couldn't know then.

Dealing with life as it is right now, with all of the changes that have occurred, requires a great deal of gentleness with yourself. I believe therapy could be very useful to help you work through these changes. Either way, it's important not to ignore what's going on in hopes all will work itself out. Taking that option interferes with emotional wellbeing.

Body, What it Does or Doesn't Do Now

Men don't seem as bothered with physical changes, though some definitely are. My work with men in psychotherapy sessions tends to revolve even more around:

Can I still have sex in the way I want to?

Can I still work to support my family?

Can I drive?

Can I eat what I want to eat?

Can I fix what needs to be fixed?

When medical treatment has brought changes in these areas, men understandably get angry, frustrated, and depressed. Many are "done" with communicating and being actively involved with life.

Emotional wellbeing has walked out the door with little opportunity of returning until some sort of intervention takes place. But in our society we don't particularly open the door to men for therapy, support groups, intimate conversations with others about thoughts and feelings. Men often suffer in silence and helplessness.

That must change. Men also need:

Psychotherapy

Support groups

Good friends to talk with about thoughts and feelings

Community, state, and national resources

Clearly, medical treatment does bring body changes, and sometimes they're permanent. It's essential to grieve the loss and process how to live now without being able to do what you once could.

Self Care

Self care is critical for both cancer patient and caregiver. This topic is constantly covered in every article I read for caregiving and less so for patients. Yet, from my psychotherapy experience, usually neither of them make self care a top priority. And when you choose not to, you begin to "lose" pieces of yourself. Think about a plant. When it's not watered, it begins to lose leaves. As it is deprived of more water, more leaves are lost, until it finally dies.

We aren't taught about the importance of self care in our society. But interestingly, we are taught about being selfish. Selfish is usually translated as taking care of yourself when you are "supposed" to constantly be taking care of others. If you're very, very lucky and have taken care of everyone else's needs, you might get a few crumbs of time for self care. Or if it's Mother's Day, Father's Day, your birthday, you have some leverage to do something for yourself.

That must change in order to maintain emotional wellbeing. And in my professional opinion, an occasional massage, golf day, manicure, go fishing time, happy hour is not enough. Instead it should be daily self care.

Defining self care for the sake of our conversation is taking care of mind, body and emotion.

Self Care Suggestions:

Surround yourself with beauty, color, plants, music you love.

Take time to love and play with your cherished pets.

Do what you love, what brings you joy, such as:

    Painting

    Sewing

    Building something

    Creating a creation

    Singing

    Reading

    Baking

    Writing

    Coloring a picture

    Knitting

    Working a crossword puzzle

    Coffee with a friend

    Tea with family members you love to be around

    Organizing

    Playing a game

Going through cookbooks to gather recipes

Watching a movie

Daydreaming

Walking

Self care is nothing more than establishing a new habit. It's a commitment you make to yourself and time you carve out for yourself every day. No excuses.

Make a note what you did each day on your calendar. Encourage yourself and others to take time for self care. Feeding the self with care brings tremendous emotional wellbeing.

Relationship Changes

One of the topics often brought up in psychotherapy deals with relationship change. It's confusing when friends that were best friends are now not "showing up" emotionally or physically to help out. Similarly, acquaintances or friends not expected to "show up" do.

Additionally, you may find your thoughts and feelings about some friendships change. What you shared together is no longer of interest or being together is now uncomfortable because your friend doesn't "get" where you're coming from. Or perhaps it's vice versa.

Understand that this is normal. Because cancer is a big deal, it can change how you feel and what you think about many things. It can also change how people relate to you.

Regardless, friends are an important part of enhancing emotional wellbeing. Sometimes, cancer brings a need for new friends.

Emotional Wellbeing Toolbox

As we discussed in Section One on Cancer Diagnosis, an emotional wellbeing toolbox is definitely a valuable resource for keeping everything organized in one place If you don't already have a suitable container and don't want to spend valuable time shopping for one, there are some available on my website at www.canceremotionalwellbeing.com.

In this toolbox you include your binder which holds:

Questions and answers from doctor appointments

Insurance receipts

Updated list of medications

Pamphlets of information on cancer, support groups, etc

Business cards from doctors, labs, etc.

Notepad

Your journal

Relaxation CD's

Helpful quotes, affirmations

Things that are very meaningful to you such as the little red heart your granddaughter gave you, the dollar you found in the grass that someone had written the word "heal" on, the orange shell you found last summer on the beach.

OVERWHELM:
TOOLS FOR COPING

Every single cancer patient, family member, or caregiver I've spoken to, both professionally and personally, "gets" overwhelm. Medical treatment and overwhelm go together like a hand in glove. Overwhelm comes because you're always dealing with the "unknown" and changes are being made as needed to address whatever is going on. These changes include what the body is experiencing such as pain, fatigue, weight gain, and the resulting emotions such as anxiety, confusion, dread, anger, depression—which define overwhelm. Additionally, you and your support system are dealing with life in general at the same time: family members, kids, bills, work, household concerns, etc.

The Merriam-Webster online dictionary states overwhelm is "to affect (someone) very strongly and to cause (someone) to have too many things to deal with."

Overwhelm is clearly a normal feeling and one that certainly can't be eliminated, no matter how much you'd like it to just go away. So instead, focus on managing overwhelm.

List of Tools to Cope With Overwhelm

CHOOSING TO 'ACCEPT' OVERWHELM
Choice rules! Making the choice

ONE THING AT A TIME
List it and follow your lead

GET VERY GOOD WITH REFRAMING
An easy skill to learn

SET BOUNDARIES
Establishing clarity with family and friends

TAKE NOTES
Tracking overwhelm

WHEN OVERWHELM TAKES OVER
How to pull yourself back

REDUCE THE NUMBERS
Actions you can take

GETTING INFORMATION
Capture what others advise

FOCAL POINT
Have this ever-ready!

QUIET THE FEAR
Embracing your power

REPLENISH YOURSELF
Determining what works for you

YOUR SLEEP
Getting it

YOUR FOOD
Eating well

EXERCISE
What can you do?

PSYCHOTHERAPY
Got your back for overwhelm

SUPPORT GROUPS
Yes, really!

YOUR FRIEND, PASTOR, MENTOR
What you can set up

RECORD IT
Gentle reminders you need now

KEEP IT SIMPLE
One word takes it

Explanation of Tools to Use for Soothing Overwhelm

CHOOSING TO 'ACCEPT' OVERWHELM

Overwhelm is a powerful emotion that has the potential to "take you over," but it doesn't have to. Your power is in realizing overwhelm typically comes with medical treatment, so you're not caught off guard. Just acknowledging overwhelm puts you in charge.

Thoughts like: "Oh there you are again." "Geez, I see you creeping up getting stronger." "I know you're there, that's okay," will keep you from getting into an emotional battle with overwhelm.

ONE THING AT A TIME

By its very nature, overwhelm gets out of control since the feeling is based on *too much*. If you can take out a piece of paper or use your phone to list the parts of what's happening in your life right now, you'll begin to manage overwhelm.

For example, first list your thoughts, keep it simple, make abbreviations:
Mom's Birthday...what to get, how to get it, when and how to get it to her. Family expecting me to come for birthday cake, don't feel like it, but don't want her to know, I do want to go.

Getting bone scan...do they/I think the cancer has spread? Maybe it has...then what am I/are we going to do? I really don't want to do this. Why is this happening? Why can't they tell me the results right after it, why do I have to wait to know, I really need to know now.

Picking up the kids from school...I know I could ask my neighbor Pat to do it. But I can't, the kids are worried. I have to act like everything's okay, but it's not, I'm not. It's important to me to get my kids from school when I can.

Why doesn't insurance cover the medication the doctor prescribed? Why is that nurse calling me to tell me that? Really, Insurance Company, does your dad/sister/brother/child have cancer...I pay good money for the insurance. Don't deny me the meds ordered. Ridiculous. Once again I have to make a call...I don't have energy for this.

Then, quickly make a new list with what's necessary to do. If you can, leave the emotion on the original list.

For example:

> Mom's Birthday
>> *get gift*
>> *go to party, limit to 1 hour*
>
> Bone Scan
>> *schedule*
>> *go to appointment*
>> *get results*
>
> Get Kids from School
>> *be there at 3*
>> *ask about their day*
>> *tell them how important it is to me to pick them up*
>> *let them know I need to rest soon after we get home*
>
> Insurance
>> *I will call them or I will ask spouse/partner/care-giver to call*

One page holds the thoughts that inspire overwhelm. You note what you feel. The other page is a set of facts that keeps you focused on exactly what you will do. Basically, it's a plan, it's black and white, mapping your next steps. It's a simple strategy, but a powerful one.

GET VERY GOOD WITH REFRAMING

A tool often used by therapists is called reframing. Look at a picture on your wall. Think about unhooking it from the wall, taking the frame off and putting a new one on it. When you apply that concept to what you're thinking about, it's giving your thought a new perspective.

For example:

Before Reframe:

"I only want to see that one nurse practitioner. I've been told the other one rushes through the visit. Ugh, I've just been told the one I want to see isn't here today."

After Reframe:

"Maybe what I've been told is wrong. Maybe this other nurse practitioner will take her time and listen to my questions. I won't know for sure until I've had an appointment with her."

Before Reframe:

"I can't sleep. I'm so tired of being so tired every single night and staying awake all night long."

After Reframe:

"I wonder if I could somehow sleep better if I changed some things about bedtime. Tonight I'm listening to the relaxation CD before I try to sleep and before that I'm putting quiet music on to clear my thoughts. I always seem to get in bed thinking about everything, which plays havoc with getting to sleep and staying asleep. I've decided to leave my thoughts in the den tonight. I can pick them up in the morning."

SET BOUNDARIES

For many, setting boundaries with people you love isn't very easy to do. However it's a skill you can learn and, especially when dealing with cancer, one that will come in handy. In fact, boundary setting is essential for boosting wellbeing.

Examples:

> You're a caregiver and your loved one wants your complete attention. You know how important it is for you to take some time out each day to re-charge. Several of your friends have volunteered to take turns staying a couple of hours each day so you can have time for self care. But your loved one refuses to consider this idea at all.

> You decide to set boundaries, knowing your loved one enjoys these friends and that everything will go smoothly while you're away. You announce, "Day after tomorrow, Jane is coming over from 10-12 to stay with you. It's important for me to take care of myself so I can give you the best care." And then, Caregiver, follow through.

> Every single weekend, all weekend long, family members and friends come for a visit. You spent all week long trying to recover, in addition to healing from surgery. No one asked and no one seemed to notice how tired you were.

> One day soon after the weekend you decided to call each one, tell them how much you love them, and let them know you'd like company only for an hour on Saturday between 2 and 3. You even asked your best friend to be there in case your family and friends decided to come early and stay late. He agreed to moni-

tor the situation and hold everyone to the timeframe you set up.

Respecting yourself is vital within cancer and caregiving. Trying to please others, worrying what others will think, and pushing yourself to do more sucks precious, needed energy. Expect when you set boundaries, if you've not done this before, for people to 'push back,' trying to get you to change your mind, or worse, ignoring the boundary. Be clear and stand by your decision. And, if needed, ask for help to maintain the set boundary.

TAKE NOTES

Get out your notepad and write down answers to these questions:

What specifically overwhelms you the most?

List several things and then rank them from most overwhelming to least overwhelming.

Can you take any action(s) to decrease overwhelm in conjunction with each thing listed?

You could explore other dimensions of overwhelm like:

> Time of day you're bothered the most
>
> Particular person/people that keep overwhelm churning
>
> Patterns of behavior that continually set up overwhelm

Learning everything you can about what in particular overwhelms you helps to point out answers for coping with it more effectively.

WHEN OVERWHELM TAKES OVER

Sometimes overwhelm just gets out of hand, even before you know what's happening. When that's the case, STOP. Take a break for a little while, choosing something soothing to do that will interrupt overwhelm.

If you're getting chemo and scary thoughts keep coming, put your earphones on and plug in to some beautiful music.

If your son calls every day for money, you're worried about paying your own bills, your daughter just totaled her car and your best friend just called to tell you about her 'bad day,' piling on even more overwhelm, take a time out. Stop everything and do something you find calming such as pet your sweet, quiet dog, get a cup of warm coffee, or look at your favorite magazine.

REDUCE THE NUMBERS

Think about an overwhelm scale. Check in with yourself, determine where are you on a scale of 1-10 – with 1 representing low overwhelm and 10 representing over-the-top overwhelm. Take that number and move it down! What tiny little action or big action could you take this very minute to move that overwhelm number down? And then what action could you take to move it down another number or two?

Observe, too, what works and what doesn't. You may decide to take a few notes, so the next time you're working on reducing your overwhelm numbers, you have some effective ideas.

GETTING INFORMATION

You can learn a lot by asking your medical team specific informational questions. You can learn even more by asking:

"If you were in my shoes, what would you do?"

OR

"If I was your daughter/son/best friend...insert appropriate term...what would you advise her/him to do?"

These questions personalize the information asked for. It's helpful to know the advice that would be given to a family member or someone close to him or her. But, in the end, you *always* have the final decision. You cannot hand over your power and just "do" whatever is said.

This question should be reserved for when you really want to get some advice, when you feel stuck as to how to move forward. It's therefore used when appropriate, not every time you have a question.

Your medical team may choose not to answer the question and they certainly have that right. If she/he doesn't feel comfortable answering, let that be okay. Move on.

FOCAL POINT

When doing a standing pose in yoga, the instructor often suggests finding a place on the wall to stare at in order to have a focal point so you keep your balance.

Similarly, with overwhelm, you want to have a focal point you can move your concentration to in order to disrupt 'overwhelm thoughts.'

For example, when you notice you are feeling overwhelmed:

Stare at your ring. Look at its shape, color, how it fits on your finger, etc.
Look at an object in the room like the light switch. How many switches are there, one, two, or three? What color is the light switch? Is the little screw that holds it in place painted? Focus on every single detail.

Pick a focal point, anything you choose, to get very interested in concentrating on. Then, put all of your attention on it. You can't feel overwhelmed and be concentrating on something else at the same time. We aren't biologically wired that way.

QUIET THE FEAR

It's important to remember that, in reality, overwhelm is just a feeling. No doubt you have so much you're dealing with, regardless of your situation, but still, it's just a feeling.

Embrace your own power by reminding yourself of this fact frequently. What feeling could you feel instead of overwhelm? How could you move yourself to feel something different? What thoughts could you think to feel something else? How will you keep yourself stuck in overwhelm?

REPLENISH YOURSELF

What is it that replenishes you even when you are overwhelmed? Write down a list of things on your tablet or on a notecard you can "go to" for replenishment at any time.

It's that story that makes you crack up every time you think about it.

It's thinking about something you love to think about like: a song you're creating, a puzzle you're trying to solve, a trip you want to take after treatment.

It's doodling on a notepad.

It's washing your face.

Whatever these things are for you, learn to count on them for freeing you up. It's a good idea as you keep finding things that 'work' to add them to your list. See how many things you can come up with, which is also another distraction for overwhelm.

YOUR SLEEP

What could be better for healing than getting "good sleep?" You know the kind I mean—where you wake up feeling rested and relaxed. I rarely hear a cancer patient or caregiver tell me, "Ah yes, I do sleep really well." Stress, overwhelm, medications, and many other things continually get in the way of good sleep. Yet we'd all agree, sleep is extremely important.

You want to do everything you can to make conditions suitable for sleeping. Some things to consider are:

> Comfortable bed and covers.
>
> Darkness with whatever light you need to see if you get up.
>
> Perfect temperature.
>
> Go to bed at the same time, wake up at the same time, if possible.
>
> Relax before bed, turn off 'intense' TV shows or movies, instead listen to soothing music, look at beautiful

pictures.

Choose not to have challenging conversations before bed, instead, have them tomorrow.

Before or just after dinner, write down everything on your paper that is bothering you. Then *leave it* on the paper. You can pick it back up in the morning. Tell yourself you are leaving it on the paper and follow through.

Regulate naps. If it makes sense, don't take them so you will feel tired at bedtime.

If needed, talk with your doctor about something to help you sleep. The idea is it's a temporary solution while you're dealing with your treatment or your loved one's treatment.

YOUR FOOD

Eating can be a challenge when you feel overwhelmed, stressed, or don't feel good physically. You may be eating too much, too little and/or eating unhealthy foods. But eating well is very important for your body and your wellbeing.

You know what to eat, what's good for you and what's not good for you. For additional guidance, many cancer treatment centers have dieticians that can help guide you with food choices. Additionally, asking other patients who are dealing with mouth sores, tastes that have changed, and other eating issues how they've solved eating issues can be especially beneficial.

EXERCISE

What did your doctor "clear" you to do? Can you walk, go to yoga, or swim? Are you following through? Many times you may not want to or feel like it. But see if you can coach yourself to follow through with exercise if the doctor said it was okay. It has continually been established that exercise is beneficial. How will you faithfully incorporate it into your daily routine?

Also, consider how you will sabotage your commitment to exercise:

> *I don't have time.*
>
> *I don't feel like it.*
>
> *I don't want to sweat.*
>
> *I'm waiting on my friend to join me.*
>
> *It's too hot, too cold, too windy, too….*
>
> *I'll start exercising tomorrow, the next day, week after next.*

We can be mighty creative coming up with excuses to get in our own way. If you think of these ahead of time, you can choose not to lean into them. Use that same "excuse" energy to exercise instead.

PSYCHOTHERAPY

When patients, caregivers, and family members walk in my door, I'm aware of an emotional "heaviness." When they leave, that "heaviness" has shifted, changed. Why? Because they had someone *listen* to whatever needed to be said. And then we focus on the "now what." What can you do, with the situation as it is, to move forward?

This is a powerful time for everyone involved. Cancer is emotionally challenging for many people. That's normal. The question is how can you best navigate cancer stress.

SUPPORT GROUPS

When support groups are suggested, many people say, "No, that's not for me. I don't need/want/like that." And maybe support groups really aren't for you. But try several out. When people "click" in support groups, the exchange of information, the support, and the relationships that are established are priceless.

> You learn about support groups from:
>
> Your doctor
>
> Your medical team
>
> People sitting in the waiting room
>
> Your community/state/national cancer organizations
>
> Your friends
>
> Your church
>
> Bulletin boards at the treatment center or hospital
>
> Online

YOUR FRIEND, PASTOR, MENTOR

Rely on trusted people to help you through various difficulties. It's okay to ask for help, for conversation, for encouragement and support. Many people are compassionate and are ready to respond with what is needed.

Sometimes you ask and sometimes others will ask you what's most useful. And sometimes it's the people you least expect that make themselves available. Those you thought would help don't/can't/won't, but others are surprisingly right there.

RECORD IT

Some people love to journal and some people hate it. It doesn't matter which fits you. What does matter is to lean in to what works best.

If you love to journal, do that. For many people, writing down their thoughts and feelings goes a long way to soothe, provide insight, and release all that's going on.

Others would like to write but are afraid of someone finding what they've written. Go ahead and write down your thoughts and feelings, then shred those pieces of paper. You still get tremendous benefit from expressing yourself, and the shredding takes care of your privacy concern.

When you do not even want to think about journaling, don't. Just because everyone is saying, "You need to journal, that would really help you. Go get a journal," etc., let that go. Journaling does not have to be your "go to" wellbeing tool. It doesn't work for everybody and it doesn't need to.

Whether you journal or not, consider keeping a list of hopeful, inspiring quotes with you, always easily accessible. These can be particularly helpful while you're sitting in the waiting room of a doctor's office, while you're resting, or any other time. Read them and, if you can, say them out loud. This helps to soothe, encourage, and empower your emotional wellbeing.

You may want to:

> Find a new quote every week that speaks to you and add it to your list.
>
> Memorize a particular quote.
>
> Re-write quotes. Sometimes the act of re-writing can bring relaxation and peacefulness.
>
> Write these on index cards you can keep them in your purse or pocket for easy access.

KEEP IT SIMPLE

Think of one, two, or a few words you can repeat throughout the day that help you feel more relaxed. Use these words to propel you through easy and hard times throughout the day. They can be surprisingly useful to rely on, regardless of what's going on at any given time.

Words such as:

> Calm
>
> Relax
>
> Peace
>
> Hope
>
> Quiet
>
> Tranquil
>
> Confident
>
> Serene
>
> Empowered
>
> Wellness
>
> Faith

Happily Surprised

Now

Expectant

Empowered

Hopeful

I can

I am

5 minutes at a time

Moving forward

DEEP HEALING RESOURCES

The above suggestions are very practical and extremely effective when dealing with overwhelm, which normally accompanies medical treatment. In addition, I have included an entire section in this book (Section 6) for anyone interested in learning about deep emotional healing. This type of healing deals with your emotional health at a much deeper level. The exercises are more intangible and require a greater investment of time, energy, and emotion, but the results last longer and are more comprehensive, affecting every area of your life in a positive way.

SUMMARY

Although you're still dealing with the anxiety brought on by the emotional shock of a cancer diagnosis, at least now you're doing something about it—deciding on a treatment plan. Doing something tangible helps emotionally, but treatment also brings additional challenges.

Making a decision with your doctor about which treatment plan is best for you can stir up a lot of emotions. This is very normal because the best treatment options available also come with a variety of side effects and not totally known outcomes.

It's very easy to become overwhelmed during this time. You have a lot on your plate. You're still getting used to the fact that you have cancer, but you're arming yourself by reading up on your type of cancer and the treatments that are considered the most effective. After you've educated yourself, you work with your doctor to make the best decision for you about a treatment plan. But on top of all that, there's regular life that has to be dealt with on a daily basis: family, work, meals, laundry, errands, finances.

Dealing with overwhelm is very common during this particular time because you're facing the unknown as well as adjusting to a lot of changes. You may sometimes feel that life is out of control and becoming unmanageable. That is a normal way to feel at this time and this section presented numerous tools you and your family members can use to deal with the overwhelm you're facing while undergoing treatment.

Sources for This Section Include:

http://nccam.nih.gov/health/whatiscam

SECTION 3

THE EMOTIONAL SHOCK OF SURVIVING

"Start where you are. Use what you have. Do what you can."

Arthur Ashe

YOUR EMOTIONS

I know it's hard to imagine but surviving comes with yet another emotional shock. After celebrating the end of treatment, reality sets in. Emotional shock comes into play as you wonder, "What happens now? I don't quite fit into my life as it was before cancer."

Shanelle was done with cancer and done with treatment. She was thrilled to be alive, and so happy she was cancer free. Shanelle brought cupcakes to everyone at the treatment center to celebrate and to thank everyone involved for helping her get through her treatment. It was the best day she could remember in a long time. That weekend, her best friend Carla brought family and friends together in a happy celebration, toasting the end of Shanelle's cancer.

But then Monday morning came—her first day back at work. While Shanelle had kept in touch with her co-workers and they were glad to see her, she felt awkward. And her co-workers felt awkward, too. Do I talk about what I went through? About what I'm feeling now? Do we treat her differently? She seems "different" now.

"You're back to your old self." But Ron wasn't. He couldn't go back to his old self now because everything was different. Ron, the extrovert, didn't recognize himself anymore. While he didn't have cancer according to scans and reports, he did have a radical prostatectomy, which profoundly interfered with his sex life, and he had to wear a "diaper" for incontinence. He wondered if he'd be better off dead.

Courtney had had a brain tumor removed and now the medical report came back she was NED—No Evidence of Disease. But would another tumor grow in its place? And what about the members of her support group who still had tumors? And what about how sometimes she couldn't remember how to do regular things—like how to get to her favorite restaurant or how to change the battery in the smoke alarm. Yes, of course she was happy to be NED. But what did it mean when her family thought she should immediately start taking care of the kids and go back to work?

Emotional shock is common after celebrating the excitement of seeing medical treatment in your rearview mirror. On the one hand you are the same person. But on the other hand, you aren't the same person at all. But people expect you to be the same. And people expect you to spring back into life as if nothing ever happened. After all, they say you're cancer free. What's your problem?

FAMILY EMOTIONS

You wonder what is wrong with your loved one? Does she not remember how awful medical treatment was? Or how together we asked for a clean bill of health—and now we have it? Why isn't he thrilled to go back to the work he loves? Why doesn't she want go out to dinner with her friends? What if something happens and the cancer returns? I don't ever want to go through that again.

Will couldn't understand why his partner Jeff wasn't getting on with life post-cancer. The doctor had cleared Jeff to go back to living exactly how he did pre-cancer. Will had been supportive, but his patience was starting to wear thin. After all, Will had taken care of Jeff, the household, the bills, and the errands. He couldn't do this forever. Jeff needed to snap out of it and get on with life.

Lauren knew her mom was scared and depressed living with metastatic cancer. She'd been given a good prognosis, but for her mom the subject always came back to, "But I still have cancer." "Yes, you do, mom. But you can do whatever you want. You have grandchildren to have fun with, and John and me, and your friends, and your garden."

His wife was diagnosed with pancreatic cancer, but somehow she survived it. Colton would never really know how his wife did it. He was so grateful. But he also found himself feeling depressed and worried much of the time. He just wanted to "protect" his wife. As a matter of fact, when Colton's wife wanted to go back to work, he didn't want her to. What if it was too much for her? What if she got stressed and the cancer came back? What if...? What if...? What if...? Colton seemed more distracted than ever. Even his boss called him out on it.

You'd think when medical treatment is over, your concerns and worries would be, too. But surprisingly, you're now propelled into the emotional shock of concerns such as: My loved one doesn't want to go back to life as it was. He's changed/she's changed. Will cancer come back?

EMOTIONAL WELLNESS FOR ALL

Countless stories could be told about post-cancer patients and caregivers who are "different now." Why? Because they are. Because you are. How could you ever be the same after cancer? That's not to deny that relief comes with the end of medical treatment. Of course, it does. But in my experience, that's the honeymoon period which transitions into emotional shock.

Emotional shock is both reacting to and working your way through psychological and/or physical changes after medical treatment. You probably weren't told this would happen, and you didn't necessarily have expectations that you would feel so different.

Coping With Emotional Shock and Treatment End

SURVIVOR. Is that the right word for You?

Interestingly, we as a society don't know how to deal with post-cancer or metastatic cancer post-treatment. We don't even have a word that everyone agrees with that defines life after cancer.

Some people want to be called a survivor because: They

survived cancer, somehow, someway. They made it through whatever surgeries, chemo, radiation, etc. that was prescribed. They are cancer-free or cancer is in remission.

Some people want to be called a thriver because: They see themselves actively thriving, staying healthy,

Some people don't want to be called anything but their name because they don't want to focus on cancer and they believe the word *survivor* separates those that are alive from those that passed away,

Does it matter what we call it? Probably not, except that perhaps it adds to the confusion and discomfort of not knowing how to address post-medical treatment for both the one who went through it and their family, friends, co-workers, etc. Regardless, the one who completed treatment gets to decide what to be called, or what not to be called.

For our conversation in this book, I will refer to someone who has completed treatment as a survivor. I do this for ease in writing and not because I necessarily choose it as the best word for addressing a person who has been discharged from medical treatment.

Changes: Body and Mind

BODY

From my psychotherapy experience, it's *impossible* to leave medical treatment, whether you're a survivor, close family member/friend, or family caregiver without experiencing some change within your body, mind, and/or spirit.

PHYSICAL AND EMOTIONAL SCARS

Scars are forever reminders of what was taken out of your body. Some can be hidden under clothes while some can be seen by everyone. Either way, they can be difficult to look at, especially when body parts have been removed. Body image is a huge deal for both men and women and it's an emotional shock to see these changes.

I have a scar running from the back of my head to the center of my ear, even part of my ear was taken. I can't believe this. I stare at the mirror and just cry. Why?

When the doctor said they'd remove my breast, I had no idea this is how I'd look. I don't want to look. I don't feel the same.

I'm wearing a lymphedema sleeve? My arms don't match? That cute little sundress? Those days are over. Who knew? I hate this!

I have to take an oxygen tank around with me? Really? That's attractive.

No one has any idea my ovaries are gone, gone, gone. My breasts are gone. Am I a girl? Am I a woman?

Oh, so I'm just somebody that can't get an erection any-more. How does that happen? Who will want me now?

Sexual changes are not unusual, including painful intercourse and erectile dysfunction. It's very normal to feel self-conscious about how your body looks and how it performs after cancer, which clearly interferes with sexual desire. You probably had no clue these changes could play such havoc with your emotions. It's the emotional shock. Talk with your medical team and with a therapist trained to deal with these new challenges. Solutions can be found that will decrease or eliminate concerns.

OTHER PHYSICAL CHANGES

You may find yourself dealing with additional body changes like:

> Early menopause
> Incontinence
> Weight gain
> Weight loss
> Swelling
> Chronic pain
> Neuropathy
> Mouth and dental concerns
> Voice box
> Ostomy bag
> Fatigue that stays and stays and stays

SCARS AND INTIMACY—WHAT TO SAY

Spouses, partners, boyfriends and girlfriends can be put off by scars and worried about intimacy:

> *I can't believe he/she looks like that.*
>
> *What am I supposed to do?*
>
> *Will it hurt if I . . . ?*
>
> *I don't feel the same way I did.*
>
> *I don't want to hurt their feelings, I just don't know what to say.*

I'm embarrassed, too—just like he/she seems to be.

I don't know if I want to stay in this relationship.

The best way to deal with all of the above is to have a conversation together about these issues. This is not an easy thing to do, no matter how close you are to one another. It requires a great deal of vulnerability and trust.

You could try saying something like:

> *I want to talk with you about my body. I feel nervous/ scared/worried/whatever you feel, but I don't think it's fair not to talk about it....*
>
> *I know you had cancer and I'm a little nervous as to how you feel about....*
>
> *I'm scared you'll see my body and be turned off by....*
>
> *It must be very hard for you to talk about cancer with me....*
>
> *What can I do to help you feel more comfortable about....*
>
> *I'm really not ready to go any farther with this now. I wonder if we could just hold hands.*
>
> *I love and cherish you for you, not your body....*
>
> *You may feel nervous about seeing my body....*
>
> *I hope/think we can figure this out together....*

LONG-TERM RELATIONSHIPS

Sometimes in long-term relationships, dealing with body changes is extremely difficult. While you're happy she's alive, while you're grateful the medical report said his cancer is gone, you have yet another emotional shock to deal with.

> *I loved her breasts, they were so beautiful. I miss them so much.*

> *He's wearing an ostomy bag. I just have a hard time looking at that, realizing he will wear this thing forever.*

> *How did we get here? Who is this person? I recognize him/her but that person looks so different. I just didn't ever think we'd be dealing with this.*

> *Why? What? How am I supposed to act like everything is just the same. It is the same, but oh so different, too.*

> *What the hell? No one could've prepared me for this.*

While you want to be very supportive, loving, patient, and kind with the one you love, you also must lean into your emotional shock with the physical changes. You can't just pretend nothing's different. It's a very good idea to work with a therapist to sort out emotional shock and body change.

Your loved one may be having a very difficult time herself/himself dealing with physical changes. It's not helpful and can be very hurtful to point out how you're having a difficult time accepting these changes.

What you don't want is for the relationship to begin to unravel or for either of you to feel alienated as a result of physical change. Therefore, a support group can be very helpful or, as suggested, working with a therapist makes a lot of sense, given the physical change(s).

DATING

Many patients I've worked with post-cancer at first reject the idea of dating again. To date would be to risk unimaginable rejection if the other person reacted badly to hearing about cancer. If that were to happen, the question becomes, "How do you not take that personally?"

So some people don't want to risk it at all. Yet, countless people who have had cancer date and, unsurprisingly, those dates move into long-term relationships.

It's okay for you to feel vulnerable and afraid. Of course, you do. It's a great idea to talk with others who have dealt with these same issues.

How did you start dating again?

Weren't you afraid to talk about cancer?

Did you talk about cancer?

What did you say?

What didn't you say?

What do you wish you'd have done differently?

Give yourself time. But then, get back out there. Cancer doesn't mean dating is over. Quite a few people have had cancer and have had these same concerns.

You may be surprised to know there are dating and relationship sites that are specific to cancer. They are listed in the resource section of this book.

FRIENDS

Sometimes you'd just like your friends to "show up," ask you how you are, validate what's going on for you now, post-cancer. Many friends, and sometimes all of them, are uncomfortable with talking anymore about cancer. After all, for them it's over and they see no need to bring up the subject. But you had cancer. And checking in with how you're doing now, physically and emotionally, usually feels better than not.

Typically the reality for them is that talking about "it" brings up mortality and the unknown, scary places for most people to contemplate. You certainly have thought about it, all of it, because the unknown is in your face. On the other hand, your friends have truly put "cancer" away. Now that you're okay, it's not anywhere close to their radar.

The take-away for you is that their non-acknowledgement has nothing to do with you at all. Don't waste time thinking they don't like you, don't love you, if they really cared, they'd.... You don't want to allow yourself to go there, because this issue is about them and their fear and has nothing whatsoever to do with you.

Within our human insecurity, it's easy to think that what someone else is doing or not doing is because we're to blame. Sometimes that's true. But more often than not, it actually has to do with what's going on inside of them.

MIND

Leah was absolutely exhausted. Yes, she'd finished medical treatment and she was very grateful her medical reports indicated the cancer was gone. But now, she had no idea how to keep up with work and take care of her husband and three young children.

Her husband had been supportive, running the kids to daycare and ball practice. He shopped for groceries, cooked, and cleaned. The kids made her cards and little gifts while she was recovering. Her boss had been supportive, asking others to take care of her work while she was out. Leah couldn't have asked for more.

So how is it now, two weeks back at work, she doesn't remember all of the things her boss asked her to include in the report? Leah had done these reports for several years. Her boss singled her out to do them because her boss said she completed them better than anyone else. On top of that, Leah's husband suddenly had to go out of town, leaving her to take care of the kids, which meant making meals, helping with homework, and taking them to after school activities. How did she do it before cancer?

When was her son's friend's birthday party? Why couldn't she make dinner while talking on the phone to her co-worker about the meeting tomorrow?

Leah wanted to scream, but she couldn't. Instead, she was so angry with herself, tears flew down her face as she cleaned the kitchen counters. She didn't want the kids to see. That would add even more to her frustration about something she couldn't explain to herself, let alone them. Chemo brain. She had heard of it, knew people with it, but she didn't have time for it.

Caitlyn and Rachel had been in a committed relationship for

15 years. A year ago, Caitlyn finished treatment for ovarian cancer. She had beat the odds and felt very blessed. Rachel felt the same, except she couldn't understand why Caitlyn didn't take care of things like she did before cancer. Things like paying bills on time, shutting the garage door when she drove out, or remembering when she last fed the cat.

They had the same conversation over and over again, with Caitlyn agreeing to remember things, take care of what need-ed to be taken care of.

Rachel felt impatient. After all, the doctor had released Cait-lyn and although she knew of chemo brain, shouldn't it be over by now? Caitlyn said she felt well, and she looked good and seemed to have her energy back. They had fun together again, life was good, but....

Jack had had his consulting business for years. He was a skilled architect, well known for his work. Jack was diag-nosed with melanoma, went through treatment, and now has chemo brain.

Jack notices he can't remember clients' projects when they call to ask a question. Jack notices when he tries to recall his pin number or his cell phone pass code. Jack's wife notices when she asks him questions like: Did you call the plumber and tell him about the shower leak and the dishwasher not cleaning well? When is the plumber coming?
Jack is sure he called the plumber...but when was he coming? Did he ask him about the shower and the dishwasher? Or just the shower? Or neither?

That international project he had been so highly recom-mended to design, what was his client's concern about the second floor archway? Why did his employee ask him where the meeting was next Wednesday that Jack had supposedly set up?

Jack found himself unraveling quickly. The worst part of it was he had no idea what to do.

Kendra was a nurse who took a leave of absence to take care of her sister Lilly while she had several rounds of chemotherapy followed by 6 weeks of radiation. Kendra lived in the next city, three hours away from Lilly and returned back to her home after Lilly completed treatment.

However, it was soon obvious Lilly was struggling with simple tasks that had always been so easy for her. Things like balancing her checkbook, typing notes for her employer, and keeping up with her son's college bills. It became even more apparent to Kendra when she returned for a weekend visit and found ice cream in the refrigerator and saw her sister trying to read a family recipe Lilly had made many times before.

Together they had discussed chemo brain, but now, Kendra was clearly very worried. She had noticed Lilly was anxious and frustrated. She had chalked that up to being a survivor. After all, Lilly had been at the treatment center every day of the workweek for months. Of course it would take time to get back into a different daily routine.

But now Kendra knew Lilly was not just trying to merge back into life after treatment. Lilly was dealing with full-blown chemo brain.

Mind changes are often attributed to chemo brain which, according to The American Cancer Society, may include:

- Forgetting things that they usually have no trouble recalling (memory lapses)

- Trouble concentrating (they can't focus on what they're doing, have a short attention span, may "space out")

- Trouble remembering details like names, dates, and sometimes larger events

- Trouble multi-tasking, like answering the phone while cooking, without losing track of one task (they are less able to do more than one thing at a time)

- Taking longer to finish things (disorganized, slower thinking and processing)

- Trouble remembering common words (unable to find the right words to finish a sentence)[1]

According to Cancer.Net, a website that provides oncology information from the American Society of Clinical Oncology, "up to 75% of people with cancer experience cognitive problems during treatment, and up to 35% have issues that continue for months after treatment has finished."[2]

COPING WITH CHEMO BRAIN

First, remember it's quite an emotional shock that you're having a hard time with your thoughts when you didn't before cancer. It's necessary for you to feel what you feel: confused, angry, scared, worried, overwhelmed, frustrated, anxious, depressed, etc. Of course you feel any or all of these in some combination. Who knew after cancer you'd experience chemo brain, in addition to all of the other physical changes. Yes, you'd heard others talking about it, but you weren't expecting this, too.

As long as you're dealing with chemo brain, it's not unusual to continue dealing with emotional shock. In a society where we value multi-tasking, remembering details, and thinking very quickly, having chemo brain isn't particularly welcomed. Yet, there it is.

Often, family members, employers, friends, and kids don't understand what's going on with you. As you struggle during a conversation to find that word you're trying so hard to re-member, they're wondering what's wrong? After all, you've finished treatment and the doctor said you were okay. Emotional shock follows them around as they try to make sense of why you seem different now.

So you're dealing with your own frustration and other emotions while society/family members/friends are often asking, "What's wrong with you?" This makes things even more frustrating. Now you're emotionally beating yourself up and those you love and work with are questioning your mental capacity, which turns your thoughts and emotions into a bonfire of frustration, worry, confusion, and numerous other emotions.

This cycle of continual frustration on top of frustration works against remembering and completing tasks. We all know this from personal experience. The more we try to do something when we're already frustrated, the less we can push through successfully.

A good example of this is when you're trying to "make" yourself go to sleep. You lie there in bed, wide-awake, with only a few hours to sleep. Every few minutes you look at the clock, getting more frustrated that you're still not asleep. "I've got to go to sleep right this minute. I only have 4 more hours before I have to get up." "I don't believe this. I've got to get some rest. I'm so tired, what's the problem, why can't I sleep?" And so it goes, often for the remainder of the night, desperately trying to fall asleep.

Similarly, it does not help for you to struggle with chemo brain. Instead:

Write down what changes you've seen and talk with your

doctor about them.

Keep track of chemo brain changes in a notebook.

Talk with others about how they manage chemo brain.

Get information from community, state, and national organizations on chemo brain.

Work with puzzles and memory games.

Keep a routine. Staying consistent decreases confusion and increases focus.

Put things in the same place every single time—such as keys, briefcase, kids' homework and notes from teachers.

Write tasks down in a notebook or use a smart phone note app.

SELF-COMPASSION

No one can understand chemo brain unless they've experienced it for themselves. You can't help but wonder if you'll go through all of life not being able to think quickly, or remember, or get things done without getting distracted. You wonder if you will ever be able to multi-task again. Even though researchers have found that multi-tasking doesn't work well, before cancer you did multi-task, and it did work for you. But it certainly doesn't now.

While you may not feel like it, self-compassion is certainly a wonderful tool to use within chemo brain.

It's okay I can't remember X. I've had cancer and my body still needs time to recover.

Maybe I could just do something else for a little while, since trying to force completion of this project is not working out at all.

I could talk with my boss about what's going on. I didn't want to because I thought I could pull this off, but clearly it's not going well.

When I relax more, I seem to be more successful with my thoughts. So why don't I:

Listen to my favorite music.

Meditate for a few minutes.

Take a walk.

Call a friend.

Read a soothing quote.

Get some tea.

Pat my dog. Watch my cat chase and pounce on her toy.

Taking a time out, then going back to your project can be very helpful to break up frustration. Having self-compassion instead of "beating up on yourself" helps to move you forward.

ACQUIRING SELF-COMPASSION

Self-compassion is something few of us really know how to do. We're brought up to think of others first and to "push through" whatever problem we're having. While that can work to a certain extent, when you throw in chemo brain, what worked before doesn't so much now.

The good news about self-compassion is it's a skill and, therefore, you can both learn and master it. Of course, that means practicing self- compassion daily. Look for ways to be kind and gentle with yourself.

Instead of insisting

> - you finish that report at one sitting, take some breaks and you'll probably find you finish faster in the end.

> - you pick your children up every day from school, take your neighbor up on her offer to bring the kids home or agree for her to bring them home on Monday, Wednesday, and Friday.

> - the house is spotless clean, assign household tasks to each member of the family, realizing it won't be done exactly how you'd do it.

> - you see every single doctor on the same day because you're already out, but find it ridiculously tiring, scatter the appointments throughout the week.

FAMILY, FRIEND, EMPLOYER, CO-WORKER COMPASSION

That emotional shock of seeing your loved one released from medical treatment but dealing with chemo brain adds yet a new bombshell to the cancer journey. While you may have heard of or even knew someone with chemo brain, you probably thought that wasn't going to happen to your loved one. You wonder how much they can take and how much you can take. You also may wonder:

How to help.

How long this will go on.

What the doctor can do about this.

How significantly chemo brain will impact daily life and work needs.

Unfortunately, no easy answers come with chemo brain. It affects some and not others. It lasts for a few weeks for some and a very long time for others. With chemo brain affecting quality of life for many cancer survivors, research is being conducted to sort out its specific details.

Meanwhile, an important action to take with your loved one is probably what you've been doing since diagnosis—offering compassion. What is most needed is compassion specific to empathy instead of sympathy.

Please watch this short video for the difference between these two terms: http://www.openculture.com/2013/12/the-power-of-empathy.html.

Remembering your loved one already feels very vulnerable, choosing to observe changes and ask open-ended questions, and choosing *not* to be critical is most helpful to them. Here are a few other suggestions.

Listen to what she/he has to say while you're not texting, on the computer, or watching TV.

Let them know you're actively listening by saying something like:

> *"So you feel concerned about your work, not being able to keep up your pace before cancer."*

"You feel scared when you can't remember words."

"You've talked with your doctor, who believes it will recede, but you want a guarantee."

OTHER WAYS TO HELP

Ask your loved one what would be of most help to them?

Suggest the two of you could research chemo brain together, to better understand what it is and what it means.

Offer to go together to a support group or to an oncology-trained therapist.

If appropriate and wanted, work together to set up routines and systems of doing things, and keep track of chemo brain together in your own notebooks.

Offer to go the doctor with your loved one to learn more information, and/or to take notes.

Seek out other people who could potentially offer help such as a pastor/minister/priest, cancer resource centers, cancer "help lines."

SELF-COMPASSION

It's necessary for you, too, to develop self-compassion. Chemo brain is not easy for anyone and involves everyone whether you're the patient or family member, caregiver, or friend. Please see more information about this in the section above with this same title.

SURVIVOR GUILT

How is it that I survived and the woman who sat next to me in the chemo chair didn't?

Why am I here?

What did I do to deserve to be called a survivor?

What did she/he do different so that survival was not the outcome?

How do I make sense of my survival?

Why did God choose me and not the other person, or did God choose at all?

What does survivorship mean?

Now what?

I don't get it. I'm no better than anyone else.

Why me? Why not me? But why me?

I've heard these and similar thoughts from survivors I've worked with in psychotherapy. While survivor guilt doesn't affect everyone, those who experience it are deeply affected. Feeling survivor guilt is normal.

Tears, confusion, anger, resentment, and depression are the emotions of survivor guilt. Trying to make sense of cancer and why I survived and you didn't defines survivor guilt. Grappling with the hard-core meaning of life taps right into survivor guilt. It is not an easy thing to deal with and its exploration doesn't come with clear-cut answers.

But nevertheless, survivor guilt is a guilt that seems to psychologically knock on your door until you take it on. It's a guilt that can't be ignored or forgotten.

If you can, set up some time with a therapist to help you explore and navigate survivor guilt.

Other things you can do are:

Journal your feelings.

Talk with a trusted family member or close friend.

Write a poem about it.

Make up a song about it.

Paint a picture.

Surround yourself with nature.

Talk with a minister/pastor/priest.

Read about it.

Go to a seminar about it or a support group.

If you feel survival guilt, realize it's an important part of dealing with the unknown. We humans struggle desperately, and helplessly sometimes, trying to make sense of our experiences, especially one that is or could be life threatening.

SURVIVOR GUILT—FAMILY MEMBERS, CAREGIVERS, AND FRIENDS

Often you find yourself dealing with emotional shock in response to survivor guilt your loved one is experiencing. You're relieved and grateful he/she is alive. While you're very sorry anyone died, you find yourself surprised by this survivor guilt emotion. You wonder where their happiness, celebration, getting-on-with-life spirit is. But survivor guilt is normal and is an important emotion within surviving cancer.

You can be most helpful to your loved one by not criticizing, blaming, or judging.

Instead:

> Validate their emotion, "It must be really hard to see someone else die of cancer."
>
> "You seem very sad about Carlene dying."
>
> "What are you feeling?" said very kindly and gently.

Survival guilt is a vulnerable experience. Your compassion and understanding can go a long way to support your loved one through it. Remember it's a normal feeling, just like your feeling of thanksgiving.

Letting Go of Caregiving

When you learned of your loved one's cancer diagnosis and prescribed medical treatment, you rearranged your life to become their caregiver. Your life has been focused in varying degrees on caring for your loved one during cancer. But now, gratefully, cancer is over or being successfully managed. And you're free to go back to your life before cancer.

Molly took care of her husband Jake throughout treatment for lymphoma. She had considerably changed her life to caregive in the way she thought would be most helpful. As a caregiver she continually shopped for and cooked nutritious foods, took Jake to all of his doctor and treatment appointments, and focused on emotionally supporting him—reading inspirational articles and quotes as much as he would listen. Additionally, Molly kept up on all of the latest research on lymphoma, and sent regular emails to family and friends to keep them informed about how Jake was doing.

In order to accomplish everything, Molly resigned from a job she loved. She stopped going to lunch and occasional dinners with friends, promising herself she'd start back up again as soon as she could.

And then, caregiving was over—yet another emotional shock to deal with. Jake was back to work and she was not. On one hand she was relieved Jake was okay, and on the other, she felt depressed. What was she supposed to do now?

Just as we discussed at the beginning of this section, being released from medical treatment is challenging, since your life as a patient is caught up with doctor appointments, chemo, radiation, surgery or some combination. Similarly, the end of medical treatment can also be very difficult for some caregivers.

You, too, must get on with life, Caregiver. What will you do now that your loved one no longer needs you to drive her/him to appointments, to cook, to help with medicines, etc.?

LIFE AFTER CANCER

Dealing With Aches and Pains

Both survivor and caregiver (if he/she is told) worry when various aches and pains are felt.

Did the cancer come back? Is it coming back?

Did the cancer spread to where the ache or pain is?

Should I call the doctor right away?

Should I wait until the next appointment?

Did I really feel something or am I imagining it?

Feeling anxious about aches and pains is normal when treatment is completed. Definitely call your doctor if you're concerned. It's better to get the needed information than to keep yourself scared by not knowing.

Dealing With Doctor Appointments

Both survivor and caregiver alike often feel emotional about upcoming doctor appointments. This is normal. It's okay to feel what you feel.

What will the doctor say?

Will he/she be distracted, impatient, something else?

Will I/she/he need to get a scan/labs/other?

What will the results show?

Am I, is he/she being seen often enough?

Will I get to see my favorite nurse practitioner, or will it be the one I don't care for?

Keeping Up With Your Emotional Wellbeing Toolbox

You'll want to continue using your wellbeing toolbox or if you don't have one, create one. Or, for your convenience, I have one available on my website at www.canceremotional-wellbeing.com. (Please see sections one and two of this book for more information on how to create your emotional wellbeing toolbox.)

Now your toolbox is all about surviving, your 'right now' post-medical treatment. Everything that has to do with diagnosis and treatment is taken OUT and sorted through, and whatever you want to keep will be stored somewhere else.

Now put in new treasures and symbols of surviving. Maybe it's that champagne cork, the summary letter from the doctor's office declaring medical treatment is completed, or the "lucky" dime you found on the sidewalk.

Write new affirmations for yourself. For example:

> What's important to me now is _____.
>
> I am moving forward with celebration and courage.
>
> I take care of me by listening to what I'm thinking and what I'm feeling, and then I take needed actions for continuing to move forward.
>
> I am calm and confident.
>
> I am creating a new life for myself now.

Add new quotes that speak to you now such as:

> "I dwell in possibility." Emily Dickinson

> "Courage is not the absence of fear, but rather the judgment that something else is more important than fear." Ambrose Redmoon

> "Life is a great and wondrous mystery, and the only thing we know that we have for sure is what is right here right now. Don't miss it." Leo Buscaglia

> "We have to acknowledge sometimes that this moment is enough. This place is enough. I am enough." Sue Monk Kidd

And Include:

> Insurance and medical receipts for post-medical treatment.

> A list of questions you continue adding to for your next doctor appointment.

> An updated list of any medications you're taking.

> Notes that pertain to post-medical treatment.

> Your journal.

> Relaxation CD's.

> Other helpful material such as pamphlets, business cards, etc.

Creating Your Life Post-Cancer

A friend of mine described life before cancer, cancer and

medical treatment, and survivorship as moving from one world to another and then to another. Pre-cancer was a world all unto itself, as was medical treatment, as is survivorship. While they are all related, they are all separate, too.

What now?

How do you move into the familiar yet foreign world of survivorship?

What do you want to be different in this new world?

Change or Stay with:

> Spouse/Partner
>
> Religious/Spiritual
>
> Friends
>
> How much time you spend with family and friends
>
> Exercise
>
> What you eat
>
> How much you sleep
>
> Work
>
> What you love to do
>
> What you don't love to do

Keep the list going. What else belongs here for you?

Survivorship is all about reviewing choices and making new ones, taking into consideration your body post-cancer. At the same time, you rejoin your familiar life with a completely different life post-medical treatment. Merging these often feels surreal, which is a normal feeling and certainly includes yet another emotional shock.

At times you can be so excited with life, so relieved to be free of treatment, you have yourself on a "high." Other times you can feel depressed as you witness such a gap, a void between the 'medical treatment' and the 'now what.' And there are times you experience both the thrill and the letdown laced with a helpless, sad feeling. Depression can especially seep in as you realize how cancer has indeed changed things for you, while everyone else is expecting you to be the same person and get on with it.

DEPRESSION: TOOLS FOR COPING

For survivorship, we'll take a close look at the emotion of depression and how you can meet it head on. As we've discussed, no one emotion "perfectly" fits each section. As a matter of fact, depression may not be in your experience at all within survivorship. You won't necessarily feel depressed. But if and when you do, try out these tools for managing this emotion.

Definition

In my psychotherapy work with cancer patients, I often define depression as a "disconnect from life." Think about when you're around a depressed person. This person has little energy for anything. She/He is sad, tired, and hopeless, feels miserable, and is in a funk. You know what depression is.

Clinical depression, on the other hand, interferes with daily functioning and is clearly treatable through medication and/or counseling. According to American Cancer Society's website, approximately 25% of cancer patients are clinically depressed.

Specific characteristics of clinical depression according to the Diagnostic and Statistical Manual published by the American Psychiatric Association include:

Five or more of the following symptoms over a two-week period, most of the day, nearly every day. At least one of the symptoms must be either a depressed mood or a loss of interest or pleasure.

- Depressed mood, such as feeling sad, empty or tearful (in children and teens, depressed mood can appear as constant irritability)

- Significantly reduced interest or feeling no pleasure in all or most activities

- Significant weight loss when not dieting, weight gain, or decrease or increase in appetite (in children, failure to gain weight as expected)

- Insomnia or increased desire to sleep

- Either restlessness or slowed behavior that can be observed by others

- Fatigue or loss of energy

- Feelings of worthlessness, or excessive or inappropriate guilt

- Trouble making decisions, or trouble thinking or concentrating

- Recurrent thoughts of death or suicide, or a suicide attempt[3]

It's best not to put off seeing your doctor if you are experiencing clinical depression symptoms. Even if you aren't clinically depressed but find yourself feeling sad/down/isolating yourself, etc., it's a good idea to see your doctor and/or to make an appointment with a therapist.

Tools for Depression

YOUR NEW ROUTINE
Yours to create!

THE WORLD JUST GOES ON
Feeling alone

MOVE YOURSELF FORWARD ONE NUMBER AT A TIME
Easy tool for feeling better immediately

TIMING OUT
Interrupting depression, moving forward

WHAT WOULD A TEACHER OR MENTOR ADVISE ME TO DO?
Powerful problem solving ideas

WHAT'S KEEPING ME STUCK?
How to get "unstuck" from depression

WHAT COULD I DO FOR ME RIGHT NOW?
Taking care to take care of you

WHY NOT?
A gentle invitation to yourself, from yourself

ENCOURAGING YOURSELF WITH SELF-TALK
Have a conversation with yourself

MAKE ONE "ME" GOAL EVERY SINGLE DAY
The power of one daily goal

ONE HAPPY THOUGHT CAN BE IMPACTFUL
Simple and effective tool for changing depression

MEDICAL CARE
Meeting roller coaster emotions head on

EMPOWERING RELATIONSHIPS
This relationship NOW

YOUR OWN AFFIRMATIONS
Creating true statements for moving yourself forward

JOURNAL YOUR FEELINGS AND THOUGHTS
Take note of your feelings and thoughts

MAKE AN APPOINTMENT WITH A THERAPIST
Helpful for navigating cancer

SUPPORT GROUPS
Beneficial for offering support and information

EAT WELL
Foods that power you up

FOCUS ON PHYSICAL ACTIVITY
What's fun?

FOCUS ON RESTORATIVE SLEEP
Not too much, not too little

Explanation of Tools to Use for Soothing

YOUR NEW ROUTINE

Out with medical treatment and/or caregiving, in with the need to establish a new routine. Routines tend to make us feel safe, secure, and settled.

> When do I want to get up?
> What will happen after I get up?
>> Meditate/pray/affirmation/write in journal?
>> Coffee, tea, juice, breakfast?
>> Dress before or after the above?
>> Exercise?
>> Leave for work/take kids to school?
> Then what?
>> Errands?
>> Work from home?
>> Write book/paint picture/sew/knit/carpentry work?
>> Clean the house/take dog for walk/conference call?
>> Make lunch/work lunch meeting/lunch with friends?
>> Pick up kids?
>> Come home from work?
> In the evening?
>> Make dinner/out to dinner/out with friends?
>> Watch TV/watch a movie/go to an event/call a friend?
> What happens at bedtime?

Time you go to bed?

Lay out clothes for next day?

Bathe? Wash face?

Read/write in journal/meditate?

How much sleep is best for you?

What about your weekend routine?

During cancer and/or caregiving these questions were mostly answered for you, centered on what was involved in your/your loved one's medical treatment. But now, you have choices to make, focused on yourself and your family's needs. When you know what you're doing and when you're doing it, depression eases and wellbeing increases.

THE WORLD JUST GOES ON

You may wonder, "How is it that everyone just goes on like cancer has never happened at all?" "Everyone just expects me to drop cancer or drop caregiving like, 'What's the big deal?'"

They were 'there' for you or maybe they 'weren't there' for you during medical treatment and now it's as if all is completely forgotten with no thought about you having difficulty merging this new life with your previous life. This can be depressing in and of itself.

And even worse, or more depressing, is when 'they' don't even ask you how you are, or what's going on with you. A gap has developed between having cancer/being a caregiver and treatment is over/caregiving is over.... It's depressing and unbelievable at the same time. For you, the world doesn't just go on. But for them, it does.

Think about a movie that powerfully affected you when you

watched it. You were caught up in it, it seemed entirely real, you could feel the tears running down your face and the churn in your stomach. You wanted to talk about it and you did.

But interestingly, it's like these other people either didn't see the movie, or didn't have much of a reaction to it. For them, it was 'just a movie.'
But for you it was so much more. It touched you deeply on a core level.
Allow yourself to feel depression or whatever you feel. If possible, don't take their reaction personally, it's just where they are. Yes, that's hard to imagine, when it so deeply touched you. And you may wonder if they really care about you at all, or it seems as if they care less. Those kind of thoughts can blow up into:

They don't REALLY care about me.

They think I've gone crazy.

They don't love me.

I'm no longer important.

I listen to them, I give to them. They aren't giving back.

What's wrong with me?

Why can't I get my act together?

I must not be good enough, smart enough.

I want/need them to be affected on a core level like I am.

I just don't get it. How can they not see what I've gone through/am going through?

I'm so sad. I'm worthless, what's the point?

The point is, Survivor/Caregiver, THEY CAN'T GET IT BE-CAUSE THEY ARE NOT IN YOUR SKIN! They have no clue what you've gone through and they're so happy it's over. They don't ever want to think about it again....EVER.

I believe it's essential to understand their 'not getting it' truly doesn't have anything to do with you at all. It has to do with them, on a very core level. Questioning yourself and your worth is depressing. But now you can choose another feeling like compassion for them, for not being able to GET IT. Then you can come much closer to understanding that for them, "Life does just go on as if nothing happened."

MOVE YOURSELF FORWARD ONE NUMBER AT A TIME

On a scale from one to ten, ask yourself what number you are, with one being not depressed at all and ten being very depressed. If you are very depressed, call your doctor.

If you are somewhat depressed, see if you can decrease your number by taking some kind of action. Turn it into a game. "I wonder if I could move from a five to a four?" "What could I do to feel a little better?"

Distract yourself.
Where is that plane flying? I'd like to go somewhere. If I could, where would I go? What would I like to do when I get there? How long could I stay? Would I go with someone? Who?

Do something.
I feel better when I get out, especially when I go to XYZ store, see some flower gardens, or walk around the lake. Or I feel better when I call my friends, clean the house, watch sports, read, etc.

Brainstorm.
Thoughts lead us to feelings.

What's going on that I'm depressed? What thoughts am I thinking? List these out, then put them in order. What could you think instead? Make a list of these. Then focus on these new thoughts.
Since we tend to think the same thoughts over and over again all day long, a habitual pattern is formed. Repeat the pattern often enough and now you think these thoughts automatically. These thoughts can move you into depression every time.

Instead, build some new thought patterns that help you feel better. What do you want to feel? Using the old "fake it 'til you make it" philosophy, think thoughts that lead you to feel good. Think them often enough and soon, without even trying, you're 'there' feeling noticeably better.

TIMING OUT

Set a timer for 15 minutes, 30 minutes, an hour or whatever amount of time feels comfortable for giving yourself a break. Use this time literally as a "time out." Read a magazine, watch a movie, listen to some music, take a shower, pet the dog, go for a walk, sit in the backyard, etc.

The only guideline that goes with this tool is doing something pleasurable for yourself. When you do something pleasurable, relaxation results, giving you time away from depression.

WHAT WOULD A TEACHER OR A MENTOR ADVISE ME TO DO?

For this tool, think of someone you admire who has helped

you through a tough time in your life or whom you think could advise you about moving through depression. Maybe it's a teacher, mentor or religious leader. Or maybe it's a movie star, an author, or someone else. The key is choosing someone who is calm and confident, someone you believe could provide guidance.

Who is that person for you?

What would he/she tell you right now about how to move forward?

What do you think this person would do if faced with the same circumstances?

Give yourself plenty of time by yourself to have an imaginary conversation with your "adviser." In my psychotherapy work with survivors and caregivers, I've found this particular exercise to be powerful, often providing surprising answers for moving forward through emotions and/or challenging situations.

WHAT'S KEEPING ME STUCK?

Sometimes you can find yourself psychologically "stuck," similar to having one foot on the accelerator and the other foot on the brake at the same time.

What do you think is keeping you stuck?

Do you want more information? If so, what kind of information?

Do you want to make a decision? If so, what is the decision?

Do you want help with something? If so, what kind of help? Who can help?

Do you need to take action? What action?

What other questions would be helpful to ask yourself?

Simply identifying how you are stuck and problem solving how you can get unstuck is empowering. Make it a point to write your answers down. Each time you get "stuck" and all of us do, you can look back at your answers for ideas you've used before and to see how far you've come for getting "unstuck."

WHAT COULD I DO FOR ME RIGHT NOW?

Depression tends to be about feeling sorry for ourselves, or feeling hopeless, helpless, or disappointed. Meet that feeling head on by asking yourself, "What could I do for me right now?" If your best friend was depressed, you'd probably ask that exact question and then you'd do something special for her/him. Get in the habit of doing the same thing for yourself.

Depression, like other emotions, is best dealt with by validating it. Of course I feel XYZ. Follow this validation with, "Now what can I do to feel better? What's the next logical step for going forward?"

So what can you do for yourself right now?

It's important to note, this tool is not about going out and spending money on big shopping sprees, nor is it about indulging on alcohol, food, etc. Think simple things like:

Plant some flowers.

Try a new recipe.

Wash your car.

Order the book or go to the library.

Go to the park.

Get up early to watch the sun rise.

Plant a garden.

Light a candle.

Write a sweet, inspirational message to yourself.

That puppy you've wanted, go get her.

The tiny kitten the friend of a friend is giving away, go get him.

Try the new restaurant you've been curious about.

WHY NOT?

When we feel depressed, it's so easy to allow life to drift on by while we stop participating. To reconnect, get in the habit of asking yourself, "Why not?"

Why not do _____?

Why not go to ____?

Why not read _____?

Why not go see _____?

Why not take the class _____?

Why not attend the workshop _____?

"Why not" is a gentle invitation you can give yourself for bridging the gap—moving from depressed to plugging back in.

ENCOURAGING YOURSELF WITH SELF-TALK

Move yourself through depression using compassion. You could say to yourself something like:

It's okay to feel what I feel. Being a survivor is not easy. I thought I'd be so joyful and I'd just move right back into life. I am thankful, but it's not easy to be so joyful and to move right back into life. So many things have changed for me.... I look at things differently, my life has changed in ways I don't seem to be able to explain, nor do I want to explain. My family, my friends, my community expects me to just go back to who I was, but that's not who I am now. No one has been in my skin to understand what I've gone through....

Continue on with this conversation, talking with yourself very kindly. Speaking out loud when you are by yourself will boost the effectiveness of this tool. Your validation of yourself is soothing, cutting through struggle and loneliness.

MAKE ONE "ME" GOAL EVERY SINGLE DAY

Each day decide on one goal you will accomplish for yourself. Choose a goal that will help you move forward. After dinner each night, or the next morning, ask, "What one thing could I do today to help me in my life now?"

Write your goal on a note card, put it in your phone, or on a calendar that you keep with you. When you have completed the goal, write down a new goal for the next day. Keep a record of goals set and goals completed. This list piles up, providing tangible evidence of completion which brings much self-satisfaction.

ONE HAPPY THOUGHT CAN BE IMPACTFUL

What one happy thought could you think about? In our "super-size" society we tend to demand more of everything. But that's not what this tool is about. Choose one, just one, happy thought you can bring to your mind throughout the day. It could be one word, one phrase, a color that strikes you, a stranger's smile, an unexpected compliment, or anything else.

JOURNAL YOUR FEELINGS AND THOUGHTS

Empty your feelings and thoughts right into that beautiful journal on your shelf. Let go, put it all down, cut out pictures, write quotes... whatever it is that is pleasing and helpful for you. It's your journal—your place for concerns, insights, inspirations, and whatever else that speaks to you.

Or you may want to write your thoughts and feelings down on a piece of paper and then shred the paper. This offers protection from someone reading what you've written, while offering a bonus of letting go right into the shredder.

MAKE AN APPOINTMENT WITH A THERAPIST

Treat yourself to an appointment with a therapist. Why not? Why not go see someone who knows all about depression and how to help you navigate through it? What's stopping you?

SUPPORT GROUPS

Check out a survivor support group in your community or online. Some are helpful and some aren't. Give yourself the gift of finding one that "fits" you. The connection within a support group can be unbelievably powerful, once you get past any awkwardness of joining in.

EAT WELL

New recipes

Foods that power you forward

Colors, beautiful colors of fresh vegetables and fruits

Farmers' markets

Gardening

Cookbooks

What foods power you up, feed you well? Intentionally choose those.

FOCUS ON PHYSICAL ACTIVITY

Get moving. Do something—anything that gets your body going. Zumba, walking, running, yoga, soccer...whatever you want (once cleared for exercise by your doctor).

One of the first things a therapist does when working with depression is to suggest some sort of physical activity. Every day do some kind of movement which provides you with the release of powerful, "feel good" endorphins. Even if you don't feel like it, or you don't want to, or whatever the reason (unless your doctor says no), make daily exercise a priority and it will decrease depression.

FOCUS ON RESTORATIVE SLEEP

Depressed people tend to lean into sleep. Get the sleep you need, but not too much.

What could you do instead of taking another nap? Focus on doing/connecting/moving. Save sleep for nighttime or if you work nights, for daytime.

DEEP HEALING RESOURCES

Depression can occur at any point in the cancer journey. The above suggestions are very practical and extremely effective when dealing with the depression that can sometimes show up after you've completed medical treatment. In addition, I have included an entire section in this book (Section 6) for anyone interested in learning about deep emotional healing. This type of healing deals with your emotional health at a much deeper level. The exercises are more intangible and require a greater investment of time, energy, and emotion, but the results last longer and are more comprehensive, affecting every area of your life in a positive way.

SUMMARY

Post-cancer medical treatment doesn't come with a name that pleases everyone. Some people like to be called survivors and some don't. Some like to be called thrivers. Some don't want to be called anything but their name. And some like other choices. In this section, I use the term survivors for getting on with the subject at hand.

Just as with cancer diagnosis and medical treatment, surviving is an emotional shock laced with the dismay of wondering "Now what?" It's often entering into a foreign land where everyone expects you to be exactly the same. After all, the doctor proclaimed you were finished with treatment. But you're not the same. You could never, ever be the same because cancer changes you forever. And it affects everyone it touches...patient, family members, caregivers, friends, and community.

But it is you, the Survivor, who is trying to fit into this new/old world again. You, who went through treatments, scans, labs, and developed a routine around these, not to mention relationships that were established with your medical team and others. Then treatment ended and you were pretty much dropped off at the curb, expected to just resume your life.

And it is you, the Caregiver, who is also trying to fit into this new/old world again. You who surrounded yourself with your loved one at home and watched her/him go through both the treatments and the aftermath, keeping everything together as best you could. You who went to appointment after appointment, got prescriptions filled, provided continual assistance, and now, somehow, you also are expected to let go and move on with your life. But life has forever changed for you, too. How are you to move forward—step back into your former life as if cancer never happened?

It is not an easy thing to do. This chapter is filled with tools and strategies for setting up life post-medical treatment. Depression is the emotion focused on in this section—since sometimes a sort of sadness and loneliness can move in after the celebration.

NOTES

1. "Chemo Brain," last revised May 30, 2012, http://www. cancer.org/treatment/treatmentsandsideeffects/physical-sideeffects/chemotherapyeffects/chemo-brain
2. "Attention, Thinking, or Memory Problems," last reviewed June, 2013,
http://www.cancer.net/navigating-cancer-care/side-effects/attention-thinking-or-memory-problems

3. "Depression (major depressive disorder)," last reviewed March 5, 2014,
http://www.mayoclinic.org/diseases-conditions/depression/expert-answers/clinical-depression/faq-20057770

SOURCES FOR THIS SECTION INCLUDE:

http://www.medscape.com/viewarticle/813529_6
http://journals.lww.com/oncology-times/Fulltext/2014/04250/NCCN_Survivorship_Guidelines_Now_Include.3.aspx

http://www2.mdanderson.org/depts/oncolog/articles/13/9-sep/9-13-1.html
http://www.cancer.org/treatment/treatmentsandsideeffects/emotionalsideeffects/anxietyfearanddepression/anxiety-fear-and-depression-depression

SECTION 4

THE EMOTIONAL SHOCK OF METASTASIS, RECURRENCE AND LATE EFFECTS

"If you're going through hell, keep going."

Winston Churchill

Emotional shock filled with disbelief and thoughts of 'This is a nightmare!' illustrates metastasis, recurrence and late effects. How could any of these happen, especially now after you've already gone through so much. You wonder how it's even possible to cope, to move forward. But you do. You somehow, someway go on—just as you did when you were first diagnosed.

Metastasis and recurrence will be explored in the first part of this section, followed by late effects. Roller coaster emotions accompany these developments, just like they accompanied diagnosis, treatment, and survival. In my experience, anger and despair are particularly pertinent and will be singled out and examined in detail.

Definition of Metastasis and Recurrence

When you have metastatic cancer, the tumor has spread from the original location to another location in the body— often, but not always, to the lungs, bones, or liver. Metastatic cancer tends to be referred to as a chronic disease by many doctors and is usually considered incurable. Medical care is focused on managing the tumor and symptoms caused by cancer. Some patients learn they have metastatic cancer when they are first diagnosed. Recurrence is similar to metastatic cancer. Local recurrence is cancer returning to where it originally began. Distant recurrence is cancer traveling to another place in the body.

YOUR EMOTIONS

Nothing can prepare you to hear the words... "cancer is back," even if you suspected it. Roller coaster emotions take your breath away as you try to listen to what the doctor is saying about scan and test results. Just as "time stopped" with the initial diagnosis, a similar reaction comes with the new one. Your mind automatically shuts down to protect itself, so you can't "hear" the plan for how to treat it.

Connie expected good news. The nurse practitioner expected good news. The doctor expected good news. But these expectations were immediately shattered as the doctor began reviewing the CT scan results with her. The cancer had metastasized to her bones and liver. She couldn't understand how this could happen after having a double mastectomy and being cancer-free for a number of years.

Mason knew something was wrong while listening to a voice mail from the doctor's office asking him to schedule an appointment. He noticed sweat was dripping onto the phone as he tried to find the number to call. He had just returned to work six months ago after chemo and radiation to treat bladder cancer. Now what? Was he dying? He had just proposed to Mackenzie, and they were planning to get married next year....

Sam and his partner James had worried for weeks about a mole on Sam's back. They looked at it almost every evening, wondering if cancer had come back. But it had been six years since Sam had been treated for melanoma. Surely it couldn't be back. Finally, they convinced themselves to have it checked out and the biopsy result indicated it had returned.

Coping With Metastasis and Recurrence

You need time to cope with the news of metastasis and recurrence. Give yourself that time, even if it's only a few hours, or a few days. Your thoughts and emotions need time to settle down some before you begin medical treatment.

Go hiking.

Sit at your kitchen table.

Call your best friend.

Play your favorite music.

Go for a drive in the country.

Take a warm shower.

Walk the beach.

Lie down.

Sit in your backyard.

Run.

Scream.

Go see your therapist.

Write in your journal.

Pray.

Hit a punching bag.

Take your time. While getting started on treatment is important, you've just re-entered a state of emotional shock. Give yourself permission to "take in" this in-your-face development so you have the necessary emotional energy to move forward.

FAMILY EMOTIONS

You had made it past cancer with your loved one, or so you thought. Life had finally returned to normal, whatever that is. But then you hear of more cancer. Life comes to a screeching halt in the moment as you try to figure out what to do. But right now you, too, are in the middle of emotional shock. Nothing quite makes sense. It's surreal to be back here again, facing metastasis or recurrence with your loved one.

Carson worked in the oil fields. He worked long hours, coming home exhausted at the end of the day. But he liked what he did. It was good money and it kept food on the table. His wife Ruby had had colorectal cancer and she'd recovered. He didn't spend much time thinking about it anymore. But what a shock one night to learn Ruby had cancer in her lungs now. It made no sense to him. Carson wasn't a crier, yet tears were flying down his cheeks. He had been absolutely certain his wife was just fine.

Maya and Lucy, sisters, knew cancer could recur. They had often talked about what they'd do if it happened. And now it had. Their brother, David, was dealing with recurrence of prostate cancer. Devastated, they tried to remember conversations and how they would handle recurrence. But now worry, confusion, and overwhelm brought any practical thinking to a complete stop.

Alice had taken care of her mom, Ethel, for 18 months. She took her to continual doctor appointments, chemo appointments, and radiation appointments. Before that, it was helping her cope with surgery. Alice had recently returned to work and made the adjustments of her mom living independently. An engineer, Alice found herself happy to be back, working on a big project that required much expertise. And then, out of the blue, her mom called to tell her the cancer was back. What was she supposed to do now? How could she fix this?

Coping

How are you to cope when you can't get past emotional shock? You had convinced yourself, your loved one, and everyone else metastatic cancer wouldn't be an issue. You had prided yourself on doing extensive research and carefully watching your loved one, believing he/she had moved past the likelihood of recurring cancer. But now, results from scans and tests show something different.
You have no idea what to do or how to get through this yet

again. No one signed up for this—not you and not your loved one. You, too, must give yourself a 'time out' to allow thoughts and feelings to catch up with your loved one's new physical developments. Before treatment decisions are made, take the needed time, as much as you can, to:

'Talk it out' with your best friend, pastor/minister/priest, therapist.

Write down what's going on inside you. You can shred it later if you want to.

Do physical exercise to release emotion.

Sit silently and meditate in the most beautiful, quiet place you can find.

Paint, draw, and sketch your thoughts and feelings.

Bring 'soothing' into whatever you're doing—such as warm soup, favorite colors, a soft blanket.

Surround yourself with beauty: flowers, quiet music, nature.

EMOTIONAL WELLNESS FOR ALL

Swirling Thoughts

Are you kidding me? Why?

Is this it?
Am I dying? Is he/she dying?

How will I get through this?

How will I as a caregiver and family member get through this?

What happens now?

Why me?

I'm exhausted.

What have I done to deserve this?

Did the doctor screw up?

If I/we did everything asked of us during treatment, why?

Life was finally settling down again post-cancer. Why now?

I knew this was going to happen.

Thoughts such as these multiply quickly until you're so caught up and distracted by them, you find yourself seemingly powerless to move forward. But these are normal thoughts and it's okay to allow yourself to think them. You're reacting to new information—details you never, ever wanted to hear. You're trying to make sense of what's happened and explain it to yourself. You want to understand. This is normal.

Emotions, Emotions, and MORE Emotions

In Section 1 we talked about emotions being like little children. (Please refer to Section 1 for additional discussion on this topic.) You can try to will them away, but they don't leave you alone. You may be feeling one or any combination of:

Terrified	Numb	Shaken
Worried	Shocked	Outraged
Rattled	Dread	Panicked
Angry	Resentful	Betrayed
Mistrustful	Despair	Irritated
Bewildered	Apprehensive	Hesitant
Confused	Hopeless	Overwhelmed

These, or other feelings, are normal. You feel what you feel.

Our society hasn't been particularly good with accepting emotions. People are often considered stronger if they don't display emotions. But emotions go hand-in-hand with life experiences. That doesn't mean you can't manage them. It does mean they are an intrinsic part of you.

The best way to work with emotions is to notice what you feel, feel the emotion, and validate it. "Of course I feel_____." If you ever feel suicidal, with plans to act on that feeling, please see your doctor, tell someone, or call 911. Sometimes emotions can become overpowering and too challenging to deal with alone.

In general, we get along with our emotions just fine. Once validated, you can determine what action you want to take for soothing and helping yourself feel better. You could ask yourself, "Is this emotion helping me move forward, or is it moving me backward?" Then you could take an action to move yourself forward.

For example, recurrence has happened.

You feel terrified. "Of course I feel terrified." The emotion is validated.

Is this emotion moving you forward or backward?

"It's moving me forward. I know this because feeling very scared will help me take whatever action I need to take to meet metastasis or recurrence head on." "First, I will work with soothing the feeling of being terrified. Next, I will make a determination of my options for treatment after talking with the doctor. And then I will choose what makes the most sense to me."

Of course, some people choose to use complementary and alternative medicines alone or in conjunction with tradition-al medical treatment. This is a group of health approaches which includes: tai chi, meditation, biofeedback, herbs, sup-plements, etc. (For more information, please see Section 2.)

Consider an example of moving backward:

Recurrence has happened.

You feel much panic, like you're frozen. "Of course I feel pan-icked." The emotion is validated.

Is this emotion moving you forward or backward?

"It's moving me backward. I know this because I don't want to move. I'm taking shallow breaths. I feel like a deer in head-lights—frozen."

What could you do to turn this around, to feel better, to move forward?
You could think: "I'm panicked because I'm feeling over-

whelmed. Maybe I could work with deepening my breathing, beginning to take longer and slower breaths. I know that my body can't be panicked at the same time it's relaxed. And while I can't necessarily relax right now, I can change my breathing so I feel less panicked.

You could think: "I don't have to make any decisions right now in this minute. Maybe I could get some fresh air, take a short walk, have a cup of tea, or something else."

Now you're in the process of moving yourself forward because you are:

> Changing your breathing.

> Slowing everything down for yourself by not expecting to make any decisions in this moment.

> Choosing a soothing action/s to take.

> Talking yourself through with gentle coaching.

You truly can become very skilled with moving forward, through validation, identifying thought patterns that aren't helpful, and taking soothing actions or choosing actions that do move you forward. (For additional tools, please see the tools for Overwhelm in Section 2.)

So, How Did This Happen to Me / Her / Him?

When you can finally get past initial thoughts and emotions, your focus may fixate on how this could've happened...again. While you knew it was possible and you worried about various aches and pains, this certainly wasn't the outcome you 'really' thought would come about. You went to all of your follow-up medical appointments, you may be eating better and exercising more, and you probably have considered how to reduce stress in your life. But now a freight train has slammed you into a surreal place of questioning.

Did you do enough research?

Did you choose the right doctor?

Did you make "right" treatment choices?

What if you chose "wrong," the doctor chose "wrong," and maybe you should've gotten a second, third or fourth opinion?

It's normal to begin to doubt yourself when you hear news of metastasis and recurrence.

You/he/she, at that point in time, did the best you/he/she could to make good decisions with the information you had. Likewise, the doctor did the same.

If now, with metastasis or recurrence, you are not happy with the medical team you have, then you can explore other options. But, it's clearly detrimental to beat yourself up, believing you should have/could have/would have chosen differently when faced with your initial cancer diagnosis. Doing this back and forth kind of thinking will keep you stuck, feeling bad, exhausted, and full of continual self-doubt.

You can't move forward when you allow the quicksand of unhelpful thoughts to paralyze you. Choose other thoughts such as:

I have confidence and trust in my doctor. I have a competent medical team. We will move forward now together to address metastasis or recurrence.

I questioned my doctor and medical team at various times throughout the original diagnosis and treatment. I didn't feel comfortable about how the disease was treated when XYZ happened. I think I will explore other doctors who specialize in this cancer.

I put my faith in my doctor and medical team and didn't really explore much research on my particular cancer. Maybe I need to take more of an active role this time around.

These thoughts and actions focus on making good decisions NOW to address metastasis or recurrence. What happened with your/her/his initial cancer diagnosis happened. That was then. You can't go back and do anything about it, at all, to change it. But NOW you can move forward with new choices. Take care to keep yourself focused on these new decisions in the present time so as not to allow self-doubt to take over.

Now that you're dealing with metastasis or recurrence, you want to keep your focus on making empowered choices, right this minute, and in all of the coming minutes. You choose to leave behind what happened before, so as to have all of your energy intact, to take you forward with new decisions that must be made.

Anything Helpful?

Can you choose to see anything, anything at all, helpful or useful from your initial diagnosis experience?

You probably have what's equivalent to a college degree in understanding a lot about different aspects of the cancer journey.

How to get cancer information/where to go to get answers:

-reliable medical websites

-local, state, and national organizations devoted to your particular cancer or cancer in general

-support groups, local and online

How your treatment center works:

-how you can get what you need as quickly as possible

-how long it takes to get test results

-which staff members you look forward to seeing and which ones you don't

-who to ask to get things done and who not to

How your medical team operates:

-what to expect when you go to an appointment

-observed strengths and weaknesses

-what you'd like to change about the process and whether it's changeable

Insurance:

-how it works and doesn't work

-hopefully how to get answers in a complicated system

While this may not seem like a big deal, it really is. This prior knowledge of the medical system, cancer, insurance, etc. helps you navigate more easily than when you were first diagnosed and probably didn't have a clue what to expect or what to do. Now you have an established base of confidence to rely on which will serve you well moving forward.

What Would Be the Most Helpful to You Now?

What do you need to help you get through this? Identify specific things on paper or on your computer. Consider the areas of:

Medical treatment

What you'd like from your caregiver

What you'd like from family members

What you'd like from friends

Emotionally

Spiritually

Other

Additionally consider bumping up self-care and self-nurturing. This isn't the time to "buck up." It is the time to be very gentle with yourself, leaning into soothing activities and actions. What can you do now for yourself? Make a list of specific doable actions you can take, with the situation exactly as it is, to love yourself through it.

Not many people do this, yet this is the very time self-care and self-love are most needed. List what you'd like to do, make some choices, and follow through. Time for caring for yourself can no longer be put off. The time is now and it's needed each and every day for emotional wellbeing. This is true for both patient and caregiver.

Caregiver, it's a very good idea for you, too, to consider what could be most helpful for you. Now that your loved one has been diagnosed with metastasis or recurrence and you are continuing or renewing your caregiving role, what is needed in terms of:

Self-care?

Relationship with your loved one?

Family members?

Emotionally?

Spiritually?

Other?

Giving time and thought to how you will move through metastasis or recurrence is essential. Seeing a therapist or joining a support group is helpful. Having a close friend or family member you can talk with and, probably more important, who will just listen, in and of itself provides needed support. If you can, evaluate throughout the day what you need, what would help, and then take action to get it.

Late Effects

Maybe you've never heard of late effects. Recently it's been getting more attention medically and in the press. Late effects originate from surgery, radiation, chemotherapy, and potentially other aspects of treatment, slamming your body with additional, significant physical concerns. As more people are living longer after cancer, more information is available for research and for understanding late effects, which can occur months or years after treatment.

Body systems involved in late effects include:

Heart	Bones	Joints	Soft tissue
Lung	Spinal cord	Dental	Nerve damage
Endocrine	Vision	Digestion	Brain
Infertility	Liver	Intestinal	Swallowing Difficulty
Pain	Sexual changes	Lymphedema	Increased risk of other cancers

Additionally, issues with learning, remembering, and attention are common, as is fatigue. Not everyone who has had cancer treatment develops late effects.

YOUR EMOTIONS

Emotional shock resurfaces with late effects, while you're dealing with roller coaster emotions. On the one hand you're grateful to be alive, on the other hand, anger, confusion, overwhelm, helplessness, and other emotions likely spring up.

Steve got through colon cancer just fine, at least fine enough. He was alive, wasn't he? And actually life had become so much richer, because he didn't worry so much about what people thought. But now, three years after treatment, he noticed he was having more difficulty breathing. Steve thought it was probably his imagination since he had had a recent check-up and everything checked out okay. But he couldn't stop thinking about it, as the symptoms seemed to be there day after day. Steve was scared, terrified really, that it could be lung cancer.

Melanie was often tired and noticed how difficult it was for her to remember things. She had never been like that before cancer. In fact, she was a bubbly extrovert, overflowing with energy. Everyone told her she ought to be an actress, because she had the necessary energy and she could remember things said to her, easily repeating conversations word for word. Melanie was depressed, feeling both helpless and hopeless, because she had no clue how to help herself. She attributed the change to aging, having recently turned 51 and being a 10-year survivor of leukemia.

William had been embarrassed since breast cancer was discovered growing in him seven years ago. When diagnosed, he thought the doctor was a quack. Men don't get breast cancer. But then, after getting two medical opinions and reading a lot on the internet, he realized it was true. During his physical, the doctor heard something in his chest that he wanted to check out further and ordered an electrocardiogram, followed by an echocardiogram. William was diagnosed with congestive heart failure, which the doctor indicated was likely connected to chemo treatments from years earlier.

Coping

Disbelief shatters your reality when you learn late effects could be responsible for new physical concerns.

> *How is it no one told me before treatment XYZ could happen?*
>
> *Why me?*
>
> *What's happened to me, to my life?*

Who am I now?

I don't recognize me anymore.

Seriously? I don't trust anything about the medical system.

How am I supposed to live with this?

My quality of life has changed forever.

I thought cancer was behind me, now....

I did everything I was asked—chemo, surgery, and radiation—and this is what I get?

How could this happen now, when I just got a new job/ in a new relationship, etc.?

My doctor screwed up. I trusted him. My life's a mess.

I've looked forward to having grandchildren all of my life, and now I have no energy to enjoy them.

If I knew this was going to happen, I wouldn't have gotten chemo in the first place.

Coping successfully with late effects is constantly "in your face." Dealing with emotional shock takes time as you try to sort through what has happened to your body, your mind, and your spirit. You may feel betrayed by the medical system and by your own body for developing more physical issues.

As with all that's happened up to now, feel what you feel. Allow yourself to feel anger, discouragement, disappointment, sadness, overwhelm, etc. At the same time, it's not surprising to feel conflicted, when emotions of gratefulness are just as strong as the ones listed above.

Yes, but I'm alive.

People are worse off than me. Why am I complaining?

It was chemo that saved my life.

The doctor said I had little chance of "beating" liver cancer, but I did. I'm lucky.

That woman I sat next to in the waiting room a couple of times, she didn't make it.

I have so much to be grateful for.

I just need to think positive.

Feel all of it, every single feeling you feel on this emotional roller coaster. Expect to be all over the place with what you feel. That's normal and part of making sense of this new development, late effects. You will likely be dealing with these feelings until late effects are resolved, if they ever are. Remember, emotional shock has once again danced in and you can't wish it away anymore than you can wish away the physical late effects.

What to do:

See an oncology-trained therapist.

Work with professionals that can help you with the late effect:

Occupational therapist

Physical therapist

Speech therapist

Dietician

Take time to brainstorm what can be helpful.

Get a referral from your doctor.

Connect with a survivor/late effect support group.

Get in touch with local/state/national organizations specific to survivors/late effects.

Have conversations as needed with your best friend, close family member, someone you've met who's experiencing similar concerns.

Nurture yourself. Incorporate daily activities you enjoy doing, even if these require modification due to physical changes.

What NOT to do:

Isolate yourself from others.

Allow depression to interfere with daily functioning. It's very important to monitor depression. See you doctor if you feel suicidal, if depression has lasted more than two weeks, or if you're constantly sleeping, etc.

Allow anxiety, fear, worry to overwhelm you. Instead, see your doctor and/or see a therapist.
Stop doing things you love and enjoy. If you can no longer do these things as you once did, make modifications, find another way, or choose other activities you can do.

Drink excessive alcohol, do drugs, stuff yourself with food.

FAMILY EMOTIONS

Quite possibly you feel outraged and resentful when thinking through why and how late effects happened to your loved one. Wasn't it enough to see them go through everything that went along with treatment, including side effects? Wasn't it enough you made certain your loved one did everything the doctor advised, including taking them to medical appointments and picking up prescriptions? Wasn't it enough you did whatever you could/had to do to support, encourage, cheer them on? And now this?

Of course, you wanted to do all that you did for your loved one. And, of course, you're thankful she/he is alive, no doubt. But now, these may be serious late effects and they certainly could require you to launch into caregiving again. Or at the very least, require you to watch your loved one deal with impactful physical changes. Why is this happening and why didn't you know anything at all about late effects?

A family of four—dad Don, mom Jan, and 8-year-old twins Julia and Tyler had been living a normal life when Don was diagnosed with Stage II esophageal cancer. Life changed dramatically. Don went on long-term disability and Jan, who had previously stayed home with the twins before cancer, was now trying to hold down a full-time job in addition to taking care of her family. In time, Don was cancer-free and working again. But then, he began having significant dental and vision problems. Now what!? And how would they make the necessary changes yet again?

Gary knew he had to get help. He didn't want to see a shrink, but he knew he had to do something. He was worried and anxious about his wife Carol. Gary had been her caregiver throughout ovarian cancer. He had seen her suffer, and together they had been prepared for the worst possible outcome. Somehow she came through treatment. But now, she had developed severe diarrhea and pain. Gary had his first full-blown panic attack, and then he had another, and another. Gary was certain he couldn't go through any of this again. He loved her so much, and he felt terrified.

Terry and Lane recently moved to New York. They had agreed that once they were settled they would go see the doctor recommended by Terry's oncologist in Maine. She had been treated for non-Hodgkin lymphoma and was finished with treatment. At the appointment, the new doctor began telling them about late effects. Terry and Lane were stunned to hear of significant risk for lung, brain, and other cancers.

EMOTIONAL WELLNESS FOR ALL

When considering and coping with late effects, stress levels skyrocket. You went through tremendously challenging ups and downs with cancer treatment, and you made it through. You, family member and caregiver, were "there" for your loved one and while they went through grueling treatment. But now, you have a whole new set of other medical issues leaping across your radar.

Why was nothing said about late effects when diagnosis and medical treatment began? Because the focus was necessarily on treating "this cancer" right now. But more and more, late effects will be discussed and become the norm, since so many people are living longer and are experiencing these.

Coping With Emotional Shock

Just as it did before, with every new development that involves cancer, emotional shock plays a huge role. Time must be given to "sit" with this shock, and to begin to make sense of it, so that you can move forward, taking needed action. Choosing not to take a time out can result in reacting and making poor choices.

In your time out, focus on soothing activities, time in nature, exercise as cleared by your doctor, beauty, music and anything else that encourages emotional wellbeing. It's also a good idea to have a conversation or conversations with someone close to you, asking him/her to be your sounding board, and then if you want it, ask him/her to give you their thoughts and feelings. Of course, it's very appropriate and I recommend seeing a therapist who can help you navigate through thoughts and emotions connected to "now what" in conjunction with late effects.

Actions to Take

Find out everything you can about whatever late effect/s you're dealing with or are at risk for. Information empowers you.

- Ask your doctor.

- Get a referral for a specialist, if needed.

- Review information on trusted websites.

- Call local/state/national organizations focused on what you're dealing with.

- Check out support groups online and in your community.

- Do you have a local university or medical school in your city, anyone specializing or doing research appropriate to your late effect?

- Attend workshops and seminars focused on late effects.

Relationship Changes

Sometimes relationships change when late effects are diagnosed. Changes in relationships may happen because:

You find you've emotionally moved on—what the two of you shared has changed. For example, your friend continually talks about how hard her life is. She has a good marriage, she has a good job, she has children, and money in the bank. You, on the other hand, are dealing with lung issues post-cancer. You're both coming from different life perspectives. Now you just feel annoyed, angry really, when she brings up how "wrong" everything is for her.

Your loved one has been in the "fight for her life"—first cancer, now late effects focused on bone pain and continual fatigue. The two of you are very close, and you've helped out with doctor appointments, errands, and cooking meals. Your friend, Susie, seems frustrated and jealous that you don't want to spend time with her. She drops comments, "You like her better...why don't you just hire a caregiver...when are you going to stop with the caregiving?" You feel sad and disappointed she doesn't "get" you're caregiving by choice. It isn't about her and it isn't anything personal. But now, you've had enough and feel the need to let go of this relationship.

You've been friends for years, and now that friend isn't emotionally available anymore. You agreed to check in with each other once or twice a week. But when you call, he/she is distracted, doesn't seem to want to talk, is busy, is something. You feel hurt and left dangling. Maybe you "went through" his mother's cancer with him or helped out when her mother had a heart attack, but now, it's as if your friend has just left you hanging.

You're still great friends and you still make time for each other. Your friendship has survived your cancer/your loved one's cancer. And now you/your loved one is dealing with physical late effects of cancer. What's confusing is when you want to talk about what's going on with you/your loved one, it's as if that friend turns "a deaf ear" to you. Everything else in the relationship is thriving. This area focused on you/your loved one's medical situation is not—so much so it's ignored. Now what?

Coping With Changed, Changing Friendships

You wouldn't have predicted your friendship would change. What was rock solid is now on shaky ground, even though perhaps you still care deeply for one another. Yet another emotional shock steps in, as you question how friendship, too, could change. But it does.

It's not unusual for changes to happen within relationships. In fact, it's normal. When life is significantly physically altered, friendship foundations may shift. Think of your home. The earth underneath it normally moves—without us even realizing it—but it does. Certainly not every relationship changes, and maybe none of yours will. But know that shifts in how you think and feel do affect relationships for many.

Options:

> If you have a relationship where you talk about your thoughts and feelings, bring up how things seem to be changing within your relationship.
>
> You may decide to spend less time together for now. Sometimes relationships need some space, some

breathing room.

Perhaps you've both moved on. It's okay to let go of a friendship that once served both of you well, but just doesn't anymore.

Getting Back to Work

Sometimes, just as with friendships, your feelings about work have changed. Maybe you loved your job or you liked it well enough, but what's happened in your life with cancer has forever shifted how you "look" at this job/career. The love, respect, joy you felt is just not there anymore.

On the other hand, perhaps you already didn't like your job/career. Or maybe you really hated it, but you stuck with it because it paid the bills. But now, you just can't stay in that job any longer.

Work relationships may change too. Maybe your boss or supervisor seemed to think highly of your work before cancer, and now she seems to be distracted or psychologically unavailable when you talk with her. Your relationship with co-workers could seem different. Maybe the connection you had together has shifted in some way that doesn't feel good anymore, for whatever reasons.

Sometimes it's clear that it'd be in your best interest to let go of a work situation, and sometimes it's not clear at all. You want to hold on, you want everything to be like it was. Regardless of how hard you try to bring it back, significant shifts have taken place within you, within them, within the work itself, and you choose not to continue.

When this happens, expect to feel grief laced with sadness,

152

disappointment, or other feelings. Another major arena in your life has changed, bringing more emotional shock. You may or may not have seen this coming. Either way, take needed time to "process" change before moving forward.

Anger and despair are two emotions that often go hand-in-hand with metastasis, recurrence, and long-term effects. You'll likely feel many emotions on this cancer roller coaster. Please check for additional emotions and their tools in other sections of this book.

List of Tools to Cope With Anger

LIST IT!
Just the facts

FOCUS IT!
What You Can Control

TAKE ACTION
Do it!

WORK WITH BREATHING TECHNIQUES
It's in the breath!

ANGRY THOUGHTS
How to interrupt them!

5 THINGS YOU COULD DO TO RELAX
Right now and later!

"TAKE A BREATH"
A mini time out

List of Tools to Cope With Despair

BRING IN HOPE: SOMEWAY, SOMEHOW
just the facts

GETTING THROUGH A CHALLENGING TIME SEGMENT BY SEGMENT
Ends "futurizing"

SOMETIMES ALL YOU CAN DO IS "SHOW UP"
It's Enough

WHAT INSPIRED ME TODAY?
Discover and explore

I WAS SURPRISED WHEN...
Hope Booster

EVALUATE WHETHER YOU'RE "RUNNING ON EMPTY"
Fill up!

FOCUS ON WHAT YOU CAN DO
Find a spark!

CATCH YOURSELF SAYING "YES, BUT" AND STOP IT
Get out of your own way!

List of Tools to Cope With Anger and Despair

EMOTIONAL WELLBEING TOOLBOX
Empowering you!

SEE AN ONCOLOGY SOCIAL WORKER OR PSYCHOLOGIST
Yes!

GO TO A SUPPORT GROUP
Why not?

CONTINUE WITH GOOD NUTRITION
Eat well!

CONTINUE EXERCISING
Move!

CONTINUE GETTING RESTORATIVE SLEEP
Are You Sleeping?

Explanation of Tools to Use for Soothing Anger

LIST IT!

Anger is inflammation, a festering of emotion, likely stemming from feeling a loss of control.

I can't "fix it, make it go away, erase these physical issues."

And the doctor can't "fix it, make it go away, erase these physical issues."

Of course you feel angry! Identify and validate that it makes sense for you to feel angry.
Then make two separate lists. One list is titled "What I Can't Change," and the other list is titled "What I Can Change." Keep these available for you to continue adding items to both lists. The key to this tool is determining facts, allowing you to see exactly what you have control over and what you don't. It brings clarity, and from that clarity, action can be taken with what you can control.

FOCUS IT!

What can you control? When you feel angry, focus your energy on "what I can control."

I can control learning more about what's happening in my body and how best to help it.

I can control getting a second medical opinion.

I can control meeting other people experiencing these same issues.

I can control saying "yes" to too many activities.

I can control my choices, making ones that are most helpful.

I can control my thoughts, choosing ones that help me best cope with whatever is at hand.

TAKE ACTION

Take action. Make choices that are moving you forward within those things you can control. Action feels better than non-action, using the energy of anger to propel you forward.

I'm cleared by my doctor to walk around the block.
I'm getting a massage.
I'm gathering recipes for vegetables. I want to eat healthier.

I'm going to the movie.

I'm sitting on my porch.
I'm calling XYZ organization to learn more about recurrence.

WORK WITH BREATHING TECHNIQUES

Work with Triangle Breathing (See Section 1)

RELAX Tool (See Section 1)

ANGRY THOUGHTS

What are you thinking about?

Right now?

Five minutes ago?

Yesterday when you went to the grocery store?

When you woke up this morning?

Sometimes we think angry thoughts over and over again. The more you think them, the angrier you get. Soon you're in an angry thought pattern. Interrupt that pattern!

What else could you think about?

What would you like to focus on?

What could you think about that would help you or be useful?

5 THINGS YOU COULD DO TO RELAX

You can't be angry and relaxed at the same time. It's physiologically impossible. Therefore, take some time to lean into relaxation. This tool asks you to note specific things you can do to relax for specific amounts of time. List these and keep them handy for relaxation ideas.

Examples:

Ideas for five minutes:

>Take some deep breaths.

>Write down an affirmation ten times.

>Read a helpful affirmation or quote ten times.

>Look outside at the birds, the squirrel, the flowers, the dog strolling by.

Ideas for fifteen minutes:

>Listen to your favorite music.

>Practice triangle breathing (see triangle breathing tool in Section 1).

>Write soothing thoughts in your journal.

>Encourage yourself with self-talk (see self-talk tool in Section 3).

Ideas for thirty minutes:

>Eat something you enjoy.

>Watch a favorite TV show.

>Take a power nap.

"TAKE A BREATH"

This tool is as simple as it gets, and can be highly effective.

Tell yourself to "take a breath," then do it. It's a mini time out and is used to interrupt anger. Pull back and think about what you want for yourself, for the situation, for your relationship. When anger is getting in the way, move it over by announcing to yourself and those involved, "Let's just take a breath." Then do it.

If in the task at hand or in the conversation you need to take more breaths, do it. Breathing and moving back on course propels you forward, while anger can keep you sidetracked indefinitely.

Explanation of Tools to Use for Soothing Despair

Despair, as you know when you're feeling it, includes hopelessness, anguish, and desperation. I've heard it described by survivors and caregivers as an emotion that goes to your very core, a deep river of distress. Despair is a normal feeling. It's best to feel it, and then after you've sorted through it, move on.

BRING IN HOPE SOMEWAY, SOMEHOW

Despair is wrapped up in loss of hope. You don't feel hopeful, but what could you do, with the situation as it is, that would make you hopeful? Make a list of things that make you hopeful.
Examples:

The sun is shining.

You received an encouraging card in the mail.

Your daughter/son called.

A magazine article that talks about someone with a

major disease and how he is coping.

Finding a penny in the street.

A new medication to address what you're dealing with.

Blooming flowers in your backyard.

Keep this list beside you and continue adding to it. Play a little game with yourself and see if you can add three things each day to your list.

GETTING THROUGH A CHALLENGING TIME SEGMENT BY SEGMENT

When you're dealing with metastasis, recurrence or late effects, it's easy to fast-forward your thinking, wondering what's going to happen. A good way to interrupt "futurizing" is to keep your thoughts in a segment-by-segment mode. When pilots fly a plane, they do not fly in a straight line from Seattle to Manhattan. They fly from Point A to Point B, then Point B to Point C, and so forth in small segments. With this tool, you do the same thing. Since no one has all of the answers anyway, thinking too far ahead may quickly result in despair and anger.

Choose to stay focused on what's happening right now. When you get new information, focus on that. You may want to list segments as you're experiencing them. If your thoughts get past that segment, reel them back in. Stay with what's going on right now.

SOMETIMES ALL YOU CAN DO IS "SHOW UP"

"Showing up" may be all you can do sometimes...and that's

okay. After "showing up," put your focus on breathing long, slow, deep inhales and exhales, resulting in a greater sense of connection and calm.

WHAT INSPIRED ME TODAY?

Looking for inspiration helps increase your emotional well-being. Maybe it was the squirrel that dropped the nut, but kept returning to the ground to pick it up. Or perhaps it was the movie you watched. Or that 4-year-old child you saw on TV/YouTube that sang so beautifully you found yourself with goose bumps. Inspiration helps move you out of despair.

I WAS SURPRISED WHEN....

Like focusing on daily inspirations, looking for what surprises you on a daily basis can bring hope from unexpected sources. Journal these or keep a list of your surprises to look back on. Your list serves as a "hope booster."

Examples:

Finding ten dollars in your pocket.

A friend treats you to lunch.

You find something you've been looking for.

Someone you loved called you "out of the blue."

EVALUATE WHETHER YOU'RE "RUNNING ON EMPTY"

Despair can be worsened when you're feeling tired, hungry, or haven't taken time for self-nurturing. Think about a car. If you don't fill your tank when it's empty, you won't be going anywhere. Likewise, when you're neglecting filling your own "psychological tank," your emotional wellbeing is greatly affected.

What can you do right now to fill your tank? How will you keep your tank filled on a continual basis? Evaluate and monitor the level of "gas" in your tank often, continually adding more as needed.

FOCUS ON WHAT YOU CAN DO

Sometimes you may find yourself caught up in despair that just keeps on re-cycling, keeping you from moving forward. Try some problem solving questions.

Write down a situation that feels hopeless to you. Then write down and answer these questions:

How can I _____?

What can I _____?

This tool ignites a spark, however small, to help you take a next step for empowering wellbeing.

CATCH YOURSELF SAYING "YES, BUT" AND STOP IT

When you're seeking a solution to a problem, sometimes a solution comes to mind or another person offers a suggestion. Instead of considering the possible solution, you say, "Yes, but...I can't." "Yes, but, it won't work out because...." "Yes, but, I don't have time to...." "Yes, but, I don't have money for...."

You may not be saying the words "Yes, but." However, in effect, you're erasing a possible solution before giving intentional consideration to it.

Instead, decide to take the thought or suggestion and think through whether any or part of it could, in fact, offer you a solution.

Explanation of Tools to Use for Anger and Despair

EMOTIONAL WELLBEING TOOLBOX

If you haven't already, clean your toolbox out and file away whatever is not useful to you right now.

Fill it with new resources for metastasis, recurrence, or late effects.

Add quotes and affirmations that are appropriate now.

Put in new treasures that help you move forward, such as a shiny rock you found in the middle of the street or a letter of encouragement from your niece.

Keep a list of pertinent books and research articles.

Keep a list of self-nurturing and soothing activities you can do in 15 minutes, in 30 minutes, and in an hour, and for when you have longer periods of time.

Include relaxation CD's or downloads on stress management.

SEE AN ONCOLOGY SOCIAL WORKER OR PSYCHOLOGIST

Have you established a relationship with a therapist yet? It's a particularly good time to get started or make another appointment as you cope with anger and despair in conjunction with metastasis, recurrence and late effects.

GO TO A SUPPORT GROUP

Have you found a support group? Many people are experiencing medical and psychological situations similar to yours. You can get encouragement, information, and support from these groups. It's worth your time to find one.

CONTINUE WITH GOOD NUTRITION

Are you cooking and/or eating new, healthy foods? If not, find a recipe today and make it. Choose something simple and fast.

CONTINUE EXERCISING

What can you do to stay active? Ask your doctor what exercises you can do now.

CONTINUE GETTING RESTORATIVE SLEEP

How are you doing with sleeping? Are you able to establish a routine, going to bed at the same time and getting up each day at the same time? Are you sleeping too few hours? If so, seek out solutions by talking with your doctor and therapist.

DEEP HEALING RESOURCES

Anger and despair can occur at any point in the cancer journey. The above suggestions are very practical and extremely effective when dealing with these emotions when they're a result of metastasis, recurrence, or late effects. In addition, I have included an entire section in this book (Section 6) for anyone interested in learning about deep emotional healing. This type of healing deals with your emotional health at a much deeper level. The exercises are more intangible and require a greater investment of time, energy, and emotion, but the results last longer and are more comprehensive, affecting every area of your life in a positive way.

SUMMARY

Metastasis, recurrence, and late effects ignite tremendous emotional shock and roller coaster emotions, much like the initial cancer diagnosis. But now, you know so much more about cancer, more than you ever wanted to know. And it's this knowledge that hurls you into wondering how and if you'll make it through this time.

Moving forward, you consider your options, and you choose those that make the most sense for your body. You learn even more coping skills as you deal with anger, despair, confusion, dread, fear, and other emotions in various combinations. You do go on, pushing forward, even when it's five minutes at a time, sometimes more and sometimes less.

Section 4 is focused on how you meet metastasis, recurrence and late effects head on. It offers tools for embracing your thoughts and feelings, and for exploring potential changes within personal and work relationships. Additionally, the section examines shifts that may occur in your thoughts and feelings about work. The emotions of anger and despair are featured with numerous coping tools.

Sources for This Section Include:

http://www.cancer.gov/cancertopics/factsheet/Sites-Types/metastatic 2013 http://www.cancer.org/treatment/understandingyourdiag-nosis/advancedcancer/advanced-cancer-what-is-metastat-ic 2014

http://www.cancer.org/treatment/survivorshipduringan-daftertreatment/understandingrecurrence/whenyourcan-cercomesback/when-cancer-comes-back-what-is-recur-rence 2013

http://www.cancer.gov/dictionary?cdrid=45861

http://nccam.nih.gov/sites/nccam.nih.gov/files/D347_05-25-2012.pdf

http://www.cancer.net/survivorship/long-term-side-ef-fects-cancer-treatment 2005-14

http://www.mayoclinic.org/diseases-conditions/cancer/in-depth/cancer-survivor/art-20045524 2014

http://www.livestrong.org/we-can-help/healthy-living-af-ter-treatment/late-effects-of-cancer-treatment/

SECTION 5

THE EMOTIONAL SHOCK OF GRIEF, DEATH, AND LOSS

"Anything that's human is mentionable, and anything that is mentionable can be more manageable. When we can talk about our feelings, they become less overwhelming, less upsetting, and less scary. ...[W]e are not alone."

Fred Rogers

Who wants to focus on grief or death? No one. But sometimes that's exactly what gets your attention, because it's literally right there in front of you.

YOUR EMOTIONS: GRIEF

Grief is a normal and necessary emotional process we human beings experience. It's not something you can just skip over, though sometimes you'd like to.

Emily learned she was dying. The doctor told her and her family together. Treatment was no longer an option. Emily "knew" without needing to hear what he had to say. She had been grieving for months now. But her family had never given up hope, and they were reacting to the news as if just now considering her death for the first time. Emily grieved their grief, if that's possible.

Henry believed he would make it. He believed with all of his heart and soul. Another treatment or clinical trial would be available to him. Henry refused to believe death was even a slight possibility. But now the doctor suggested hospice to him. He felt confused and lost. The doctor had given up on him?

Leah was a religious woman who taught Sunday school and served on various committees at her church. Five years ago, Leah found a lump in her breast and had surgery, chemo, and radiation and had been cancer-free. Six months ago, when Leah went in for her check-up, scan results indicated cancer had come back and was now in her bones, lungs, and liver. How could this be? She felt mad and resentful, wondering how God could do this to her?

Evan and his wife Jo had been together for 16 years. Jo had begun taking care of Evan when he was diagnosed with colon cancer. But now, cancer-free, Evan was taking care of Jo, who had recently been diagnosed with an aggressive form of brain cancer. His wife was dying and Evan was caught up in relentless guilt and grief.

Anticipatory Grief

When a diagnosis is made indicating treatment will no longer be helpful, anticipatory grief begins. Anticipatory grief is defined by David Kessler as "the grief we privately feel before a loved one dies. It was originally called preparatory grief, which in some ways describes it more accurately. It is how our mind, heart and soul prepare for impending loss. Not only do those who are about to lose someone feel it, but often the dying person feels it too."[1]

Anticipatory grief can be a solitary, internal process marked by an unwillingness to verbalize feelings about the coming loss. Patients, family members, friends, and caregivers all usually experience anticipatory grief.

Anticipating grief and the grieving you go through is not easy. It's terribly difficult to think about *letting go* before death, but you do. You can't stop it. It's normal grieving.

"Self Grief"

Grieving for yourself, letting go of your own life, comes with emotional shock, even if you knew death was coming. It's one of the most difficult circumstances anyone ever faces. "Self grief" is necessarily saying goodbye to your life:

Your relationships with family members, friends, and everyone you've connected with

Your pets

All of the things you love like being in the garden, watching sunrises and sunsets, your favorite music, your home, your treasured books, etc.

Your memories and life stories

How Do You, Can You, Possibly Let Go?

You cry.

You scream.

You deny you're dying.

You get mad.

You feel guilty for being a "burden" on your caregiver, family members.

You ask for more time here on Earth.

You agree to try harder, be a better person.

You over-exert yourself physically.

All of these define your grief. And they are all normal activities of grief. Your emotions at this time are constant, front and center ... and normal!

FAMILY EMOTIONS

Grief is very complicated because you're faced with letting go of your loved one, while at the same time "being there" for your loved one while she/he is letting go of their own life. How much of your emotions do you show and how much of your emotions, if any, do you try to hide from your loved one?

Ellie had taken care of her father for several years. He was almost 75 and had recently taken a turn for the worse. Her father seemed to be accepting his coming death better than she was. Ellie felt pulled between how much she loved her father and her guilt when she thought about how things would ease up for her when she was no longer needed for caregiving.

Vicki and Julia had been inseparable for years. They lived together and they established a business together. Now Julia was dying from brain cancer. Vicki cried continually, at first alone, and now with Julia, bringing much needed relief. Precious time was spent reliving memories, looking at their pictures and the treasures they bought together.

Stan's wife had never seen Stan so upset. She continually reminded him that he wasn't dying, she was. Stan had lost all desire to work, to see family members, to do anything at all except take care of his wife's needs. His wife finally insisted he see a therapist. Very reluctantly he agreed to honor her wish, but only if she went with him to the appointment. Together they were able to embrace grief, honoring their lives and coping with approaching death.

Coping With Your Grief

How are you supposed to get through the death of your loved one? Where's the guidebook for that? Where's the acceptance from society that you're "torn up" inside. And where's the extra energy you need to deal with your grief while taking care of your loved one? Emotional shock wells up as you try to figure it all out. And perhaps, most of the time, you can't.

You may be caught up with various combinations of emotion such as:

Overwhelm	Dread	Guilt
Confusion	Disbelief	Worry
Anger	Denial	Lost
Sadness	Anxiety	Numb

All of these are normal "grief" feelings. Feel what you feel. Allow yourself to grieve.

EMOTIONAL WELLNESS FOR ALL

Kendra and her husband John were high school sweethearts. They had a close family with 5 children, 12 grandchildren and another grandbaby on the way. Life was full of many ups and downs, but none of these were as immobilizing as learning Kendra had only a few months to live. Each of them wondered in their own way how this was even possible. Kendra looked just like she always looked. Maybe she had slowed down some, but was she really sick? However, the doctor had been very certain as he showed them scans and explained what was happening in Kendra's body.

Coping with their grief, they decided to have a family sleepover. Everyone brought food and sleeping bags. Together they told stories, played games, laughed and cried. It was a time each of them would cherish forever.

Cole was getting sicker, losing strength daily. He was worried and confused about this new development, having just heard his doctor's recommendation to call hospice. He walked out of the appointment, sitting down in the waiting room wondering what to do, wiping off silent tears. The navigator at the treatment center saw him as he was walking down the hall. Together they mapped out some ideas for how to let his family know and how to move forward with hospice.

Suzie wanted to die with several close family members and friends beside her. She wanted to have candles lit and soft jazz playing. She imagined peacefully passing away in the midst of happy conversation and memory sharing. Then she hoped everyone would gather for a true celebration of her life at her memorial service.

Just as there is no "right way" to go through cancer, there is also no "right way" to go through grief. We don't have a formula that will take you through smoothly. Every person's grief is their own, experienced in their own way. Concern comes into play if clinical depression is apparent or if an emotion that seems over-the-top is being expressed in unhealthy ways.

Clinical Depression

Grace had been her husband's caregiver for just over a year. Together they had gone through the many highs and lows of treatment. A month ago, the doctor had told them both that treatment was no longer an option.

Grace slid into a deep depression. She couldn't make herself get out of bed. What did it matter since her husband was now in a hospital bed in another room? Besides, the new full-time caregiver they had decided to hire could give her husband the care he needed.

She was spending less and less time with her husband. She no longer answered phone calls. She had no appetite. Grace just wanted to die when her beloved husband died.

The caregiver noticed how Grace had changed. She spoke with Grace about her concern. While they were having this conversation, Grace's sister unexpectedly stopped by. Her sister hadn't seen Grace in several weeks, because Grace had told her that with the caregiver there and everything was okay. But now Grace's sister could see everything was not okay at all.

Trying Hard to Stay Upbeat

When you're grieving, sometimes you put so much emotional energy into being upbeat, positive, even perky, that you exhaust your precious energy. It's not uncommon and is a normal coping mechanism associated with denial.

This denial is aggravated by our society, that doesn't seem to accept or want people to grieve. But when death is at hand, give yourself permission:

> to feel it.

> to know it.

> to think it.

> to experience it.

> to be with it.

You can still maintain your positive attitude, your desire to find hope and joy, even with death on its way.

Grief and Anger

Trying to resolve why this is happening brings anger. Why? Why? WHY? But you can find no good reasons. You're coping with "the unknown." It's okay to be angry anyway.

Grief and Guilt

> *Why didn't I take better care of myself?*

> *Why didn't the medicine work?*

Why is she dying/he dying and I'm not?

Why didn't I insist on taking her to the doctor sooner?

But there are no good answers here. You did what you did. Feeling guilty will not change any of it and robs your energy. It's okay. Allow the guilt to subside. Fill your time with what you'd like to feel.

How?

- Focus on what you'd like to feel instead of guilt.

- Each time guilt comes up, acknowledge it… "There's guilt again."

- Then shift your focus to the feelings you want to feel.

- Repeat, repeat, repeat…establishing a new pattern of thought, one that feels better.

Soothing Grief

As we've discussed, grieving goes hand in hand with dying and death. It's normal. What could be very helpful is to look for ways to soothe yourself within the grief process. Self-care doesn't take away from grief. It helps you move through grief.

Lean into soothing yourself with:

A warm blanket

A cup of tea

Another pillow

Snuggle with your pet

Socks

Light a candle

Wear comfortable clothes

Journal your thoughts and feelings

Storytelling, Desires, Appreciation

Consider what you'd like to leave with your loved ones:

Stories

Hopes and dreams for them

Appreciation

Mentoring

Thoughts about life

Poems

Quotes

Shared conversations

All of these can easily be videotaped or recorded with your smart phone, computer, etc. You may want to have the camera or recorder on you or you may want to include family members and/or friends. Recordings could be planned or impromptu, perhaps at a family gathering.

Other Ideas for Giving

Write cards or letters

Draw

Gather pictures

Put together a package of treasured mementos

Creating these gifts is especially helpful for coping with grief now, and for having precious tangible gifts for remembering later on.

YOUR EMOTIONS: DEATH

Death usually comes before anyone is really ready. We want more time to do the things we love and to be with people we love.

Holding On, Before Death

Sometimes when you're dying, you just want to hold on a few days, a few months, or more. You want to "make it" to see your grandson graduate. You want to see your daughter get married. Or you just want to continue to be there with those you love. That's a normal response. Of course you want to "be there." And that's okay.

But sometimes, you think you need to hold on. You believe you must stay alive for those you love, because they need you to stay alive. Or maybe it's because you don't believe it's okay to die. However, when that time comes, if you can, give yourself permission to peacefully let go. You'll make your way and so will everyone else. Be easy with yourself.

Coping With Death

Death in our society is just hard for us.

We don't want to think about it.

We don't want to talk about it.

We don't very much want to prepare for it, even when it's imminent.

Many of us struggle terribly with death and dying, despite knowing each one of us will die. What might happen if you and your loved ones, together, spent some time talking and planning what you want to happen when death comes?

Will you have:

A religious service?

A memorial?

A party to celebrate your life?

Nothing? Something else?

What clothes do you want to wear?

Will you be cremated or buried?

Do you want singing, dancing, cultural traditions carried out?

Who do you want to be in charge of "seeing these things through?"

What other things do you want to consider?

Maybe you're already having these conversations and maybe you just don't want to/need to. Whatever you decide is just fine. Talking about death together, while always difficult, helps give your family members needed direction in a time of roller coaster emotions.

FAMILY EMOTIONS

You wonder how you'll ever "survive" without your loved one. You've been through thick and thin together. Your life has been all the richer because of this person you hold so dear. And now you're supposed to just let go of them. Really?

None of us get much direction on how to make sense of a loved one's death, especially when it's complicated by having cancer. Religious beliefs can offer help. Our friends and family members can be there to talk us through. But still, death leaves such a hole, an emptiness laced with tremendous emotion.

Coping

You cry and cry and then cry some more.

You get angry. How could your loved one leave you and why did cancer happen?

You smile thinking of the fun times, the celebrations together.

You feel overwhelmed, wondering how you're supposed to get on with life without him/her.

You try to keep busy—very, very busy.

You hike to the top of a mountain and "sit" with your loss.

You pray.

You journal.

You feel grateful for the time you had together.

You laugh thinking about that silly story your loved one told you.

You feel exhausted with grief and loss.

You feel restless.

You feel peaceful that your loved one is at peace.

Roller coaster emotions accompany grief and loss. On many levels you're just trying to make sense of life without the one you love. That requires:

Feeling what you feel. It naturally just occurs.

Taking good care of yourself, as your loved one would want you to do.

Being with those you love.

The passing of time.

Grief and Loss—How Long?

After the death of a loved one, grief and loss go everywhere with you. You hear a song and think of shared time together. You're at a family gathering and expect her to be there. You're out shopping and see someone that looks like him. You're surrounded by thoughts and emotions wrapped up in loss.

As time goes by, you may notice getting caught up in whatever you're doing and grief is not front and center. While you will never, ever forget that person you love, you do somehow, some way, go on with your life—in short increments that continue to get longer.

Making your way through grief and loss takes a very, very long time. Give yourself that time. While your friends, family members and our society urge you to move on, it must be at your pace. Trying to hurry through your grief tends to slow down moving forward.

That said, notice if you feel depression or some other feeling that interferes with daily routines such as eating, sleeping, working, and tending to responsibilities like feeding the cat, going to the grocery store or paying the bills. If this is happening, pay attention. It's important to make an appointment with your doctor and/or therapist to help get you through this time. Taking an antidepressant or some other appropriate medication doesn't make you weak or crazy. Rather, it helps you cope, usually temporarily, with your grief and loss.

EMOTIONAL WELLNESS FOR ALL

Death tends to be the white elephant in the living room. We as a society don't like to think about it or talk about it, unless we have to. Cancer forces you to think and talk about it. When you're facing death and your loved ones are facing your death, the white elephant necessarily disappears, because now you no longer have the option of ignoring it.

But you want to manage fear, overwhelm, worry, and every other emotion as best you can. While this is tremendously challenging, consider:

Self-care—exercise, eat well, sleep.

Do what you can to soothe: meditate, warm tea, cozy blanket, affirmations, walk in nature.

Hold family meetings so everyone knows what's going on and can share in decision-making.

Contact Hospice for care, if your loved one is agreeable, or home health if more care is needed.

Keep life as simple as possible—whatever commitments you can take a break from, do so. It's not the time to take on new responsibilities. Sometimes you may want to, as a way to cope, but in the end it's more stressful.

What else can you think of to help yourself and those you love?

List of Tools to Cope With Grief

TIME STOPS
What to do now

QUESTIONS TO ASK YOURSELF
Answers guide you through

ADVANCED DIRECTIVES
Tool for helping you clarify

FLOWING WITH GRIEF
Moving *through* grief

CONVERSATION WITH YOURSELF
It's okay to feel...

LOOKING FOR A SMILE
How to find one

TAKING CARE TO TAKE CARE OF YOU
Moments matter

"CALLING OUT" GRIEF
Gaining insight

TAKE A GRIEF BREAK
Pause it

FIND A THEME SONG
Encouraging words

ONE STEP AT A TIME
Tightrope Walking

TLC YOURSELF
Five things you can do

HAVE CONVERSATIONS
Talk, talk, talk

SEND YOURSELF A CARD
Soothing words

SCHEDULING YOUR TIME
Structure is good

TALK WITH YOUR DOCTOR IF
Grief is interfering with normal functioning

SEE AN ONCOLOGY SOCIAL WORKER, PSYCHOLOGIST
Get a referral from your doctor or medical team

GO TO A SUPPORT GROUP
Grief groups are available

GOOD NUTRITION
Eat nutritiously

EXERCISING
What can you do to stay active? Check with your doctor

RESTORATIVE SLEEP
Resources for enhancing sleep are in RESOURCES. Find them in the back of this book

Explanation of Tools for Soothing Grief

TIME STOPS

Both anticipatory grief and grieving are "time stopping." Your attention is focused on "right now, upfront, this can't be happening/this is happening." Give yourself that time to just be distracted. You may want to talk with your boss, your family, your teachers, and whoever else is in your daily life so they understand your distress.

Take time to just "be" with your grief. Cry, scream, get mad, kick the soccer ball, take a hot shower, punch the punching bag, journal, fret, get coffee with a friend, pet the dog and the cat, paint a picture, go fishing, look at the stars, plant some flowers, light a candle, send yourself some flowers, walk in nature, or whatever else that is not harmful to yourself or others.

QUESTIONS TO ASK YOURSELF

Ask and answer:

> What are my thoughts and feelings about death and dying?

> How will I take care of myself physically, emotionally, and spiritually while dying takes place?

> How can I best support my loved ones during this time?

> What are my thoughts and feelings about hospice care?

> How will I say goodbye to my beloved? When will I say goodbye?

> Do I have anything that "needs" to be resolved with my loved ones? If so, do I resolve it with each person or do I resolve it in another way such as talking with a psychotherapist, writing a letter (that does not get sent), etc.

ADVANCED DIRECTIVES

Advanced directives are important documents that let your doctor know what medical care you want or don't want to have when death is at hand. It is necessary to complete these before they are needed. Since states vary on how they are managed, be certain you know what your state requires for advanced directives. Please see RESOURCES in the back of the book for more information.

FLOWING WITH GRIEF

You cannot "run away" from grief. It's a normal emotional process and is necessary to "go through." You may find yourself crying one minute, feeling angry the next, and deciding you are just fine in the next (though you don't really feel just fine). Expect this. It's all part of healthy grieving.

CONVERSATION WITH YOURSELF

Have a conversation with yourself—out loud, if you're alone. Let yourself know it's okay to feel what you feel. Giving yourself "permission" to grieve and acknowledging what you feel goes a long way in helping you move through your feelings. Trying to "stuff" your grief doesn't work as feelings can only be pushed down temporarily. They will surface.

LOOKING FOR A SMILE

Grief and smiles don't often go hand-in-hand. Yet, taking a bit of time to smile is helpful for lightening your grief. Some people feel guilty when they smile while going through their sadness. It's okay to smile. What one thing could you find right now to smile about?

TAKING CARE TO TAKE CARE OF YOU

Find moments to soothe yourself. What could you do right

now for you? You could treat yourself to an ice cream cone, watch the little boy swinging at the park, wake up early to see the sunrise, or something else. Get a note card and write down the day and date at the top. Then, each day keep track of what you are doing for yourself. Write down at least two things each day.

"CALLING OUT" GRIEF

Find a way to learn more about your grief. For example could you draw a picture of it or make up a poem about it? Could you write an article or a story about grief? While this may be the last thing you feel like doing, when you just do it anyway, surprising insight can surface.

TAKE A GRIEF BREAK

While feeling and experiencing your grief is essential to moving through it, taking a break is okay, too. Choose a comfortable amount of time and set your timer or watch for that amount. Then, do something else unrelated to grief.

FIND A THEME SONG

Choose a song that "moves" you, encourages you, and offers strength. Listen to it! Sing it! Write the words down on a note card. Music is wonderful for soothing grief.

ONE STEP AT A TIME

Think of a tightrope walker for helping yourself move forward. A tightrope walker can only move ever so slowly forward. If she looks down, falling is a real possibility. If she looks too far left or too far right, falling is a real possibility. Or if she looks too far across, hurrying a bit to get to the other side in order to get off the tightrope, falling is a real possibility.

Grieving is like that. Grief takes its own time. It can't be rushed or hurried.

TLC YOURSELF

"Tender Loving Care Yourself" is a good thing to keep in mind throughout grief. Grief calls for being especially gentle and loving with yourself, continually finding ways to soothe and ease the emotion you are experiencing. Keep a running list in your spiral notebook of ways to TLC Yourself. Refer to it often for ideas.

HAVE CONVERSATIONS

It's okay to talk about your grief with others. Sometimes hearing yourself talk about it can offer insight and direction. Additionally, the listener may be able to offer helpful suggestions. Actively choose to talk about your grief with people who will be supportive.

SEND YOURSELF A CARD

Go to the store, pick out a beautiful card, and send it to yourself. Find a card with encouraging, supportive words, and then write some of your own. Mail it to yourself. Enjoy opening your card and put it in a place where you will see it often.

SCHEDULING YOUR TIME

While you may not feel much like having any kind of schedule or routine when you're grieving, try to keep some semblance of one. This is certainly not the time to be rigid with yourself, but having some structure can help move you forward.

GO SEE YOUR DOCTOR

If grief is interfering with daily functioning, schedule a time with your doctor. Sometimes grief can be of such intensity that medical intervention is needed.

SEE AN ONCOLOGY SOCIAL WORKER, PSYCHOLOGIST

Going to see a therapist while grieving can be of great benefit. Being "heard" is very soothing. In addition, she can offer guidance for continuing to move through grief.

GO TO A SUPPORT GROUP

Support groups focused on grief are available in most communities. Being around others experiencing similar circumstances and emotions offers "needed" support.

GOOD NUTRITION

Sometimes when grieving, people find they have no appetite, while others find themselves continually eating. Neither of these are good choices. Instead, pay particular attention to eating nutritiously, choosing appropriate quantities, even when you don't want to.

EXERCISING

With your doctor's "go ahead," continue to stay as active as you can. Clearly, exercise helps balance and ease emotions.

RESTORATIVE SLEEP

Resources for enhancing sleep are in the RESOURCES section. You can find them in the back of this book.

List of Tools to Cope With Loss

MANAGING LOSS
Memories, Birthdays, Anniversaries

FEELING GUILTY?
Sometimes you do

SOOTHING SELF
Emotional balm

WHAT ARE THE GIFTS?
Good things

HOW COULD I?
Move yourself forward quickly

WHAT HELPED ME TODAY?
Insight for tomorrow

SMILES?
Bring them on

MAGNIFY WELLBEING
How to expand it

ONE THING IN YOUR POCKET
Take it with you

THE OK METER
Moving forward on it

HELIUM BALLOONS
Concern be gone

ASK YOURSELF WHY NOT?
Then follow through

HOLD YOUR OWN HAND
Showing up for yourself

SHRINK IT
Contracting a thought or feeling

SEE AN ONCOLOGY SOCIAL WORKER, PSYCHOLOGIST
Get a referral from your doctor or medical team

CONTINUE WITH GOOD NUTRITION
Enhances emotional wellbeing

CONTINUE EXERCISING
Keep moving

CONTINUE GETTING RESTORATIVE SLEEP
Resources for enhancing sleep are in RESOURCES. You can find them in the back of this book

Explanation of Tools to Use for Soothing Loss

Emotional wellbeing doesn't mean you'll no longer feel emotion connected to memories you have or when birthdays and anniversaries occur. In fact, emotions often intensify as you remember your loved one. Sometimes you may be caught off guard—one minute you feel just fine, the next you are crying when you think about the time....

Birthdays and anniversaries are known for stirring up emotions as you remember these special times shared with your loved one. Expect this, setting time aside to acknowledge the occasion.

It's normal to feel yourself move back into grief when you think about memories or special celebration days. Be easy with yourself and lean into the emotion, allowing yourself to feel what you feel. Gradually these feelings will subside and emotional wellbeing will return.

FEELING GUILTY?

As you begin new relationships, you may find yourself feeling guilty or feeling concerned about betraying the relationship you had with your loved one. This is a normal feeling. What would your loved one say to you? Would your loved one want you to be happy, to move forward, to establish new connections with life as it is now?

SOOTHING YOURSELF

What is your emotional balm? What is it you do for yourself to enhance emotional wellbeing?

WHAT ARE THE GIFTS?

As the "rawness" of loss heals, spend some time focusing on the many good things in your life. Start a list in a spiral notebook. Continue adding daily to your list, reflecting on them. You may want to use a journal for recording your thoughts about the gifts. Some people have a dedicated gratitude journal.

HOW COULD I?

After loss, sometimes it's difficult to motivate yourself to take on new relationships or new activities. You can keep yourself from moving forward by believing too much effort is involved.

Try thinking of something you'd like to accomplish. Then think of one tiny thing you could do that would move you in the direction of accomplishing that thing. One tiny action moves you closer—a string of tiny actions gets you where you want to go.

WHAT HELPED ME TODAY?

Find a time each day to reflect on what is helping you move forward, enhancing your emotional wellbeing. Keep a list of these tools, reading them often and adding to them.

SMILES

What brings a smile to you?

Think it.

Do it.

Watch it.

Be it.

Create it.

Look at a picture of it.

Listen to it.

Paint it.

Smell it.

Write it.

Touch it.

Gather it.

Cook it.

MAGNIFY WELLBEING

When you focus on emotional wellbeing, you'll find yourself feeling more emotional wellbeing since what we focus on expands. This tool involves "playing with" wellbeing.

Imagine you're completely filled with emotional wellbeing. How do you feel? Write a letter to yourself explaining in detail what it's like to feel wellbeing.

Could you make up a song about it? Or could you sing a song you know that represents wellbeing for you? What about creating something that represents emotional wellbeing? Maybe you will sculpt clay, paint, carve, build, paint, plant, etc. something meaningful.

ONE THING IN YOUR POCKET

Choose one thing you can keep in your pocket symbolizing peace, courage, or anything else helpful to you. You might choose a favorite coin, a small heart, a favorite fortune from a fortune cookie. Or you may want to create something.

Whatever you choose, each time you take the small object out to look at it, associate it with peace, courage, or whatever is helpful for you.

THE OK METER

In your imagination or on a piece of paper, draw a round circle with a dial. Circle numbers one through ten around the dial. One is a low rating on the OK meter indicating things are not feeling OK inside. Ten is a high rating, indicating you are feeling very OK, fabulous OK. Where are you on the OK meter? Check in with yourself frequently. Maybe right now you are coming in as a 3. Could you raise it to 4, 5, or an 8? How would you do that? Think of specific actions you could take right now to push the number higher.

HELIUM BALLOON

Visualize psychologically "letting go" of an issue that's troubling you. Imagine writing down what's bothering you on a note card, inserting the folded note card in a helium balloon, and watching the balloon carry the concern away. You can also use this tool for worry, unfounded fear, overwhelm, anxiety, etc.

ASK YOURSELF WHY NOT?

Why not go out for coffee?

Why not check into that exercise program?

Why not sign up for the hike?

Why not take the class?

Why not get a puppy?

Why not......?

Sometimes after loss, you may need a nudge to help yourself get going. "Why not" is a simple question and, when answered, spurs action.

HOLD YOUR OWN HAND

Most of us are fortunate to have two hands and can do this. Holding your own hand can be very soothing, when you think about it in this way.

SHRINK IT

If you're feeling scared, worried, or something similar, imagine that feeling in the palm of your hand. See if you can shrink that feeling to a smaller form, then gently blow it off your palm. Let the feeling go.

MAKE AN APPOINTMENT WITH A THERAPIST

Making your way through grief and loss is not easy. Just having someone who is objective listen to you is helpful for sorting emotions and for moving forward. Choose a therapist who knows a lot about grief and loss. Check with your doctor or someone you trust for a referral.

CONTINUE WITH GOOD NUTRITION

Eating well naturally enhances emotional wellbeing. You might want to get creative trying some new recipes or tasting some new foods. Why not?

CONTINUE EXERCISING

Exercising is well known for releasing chemicals resulting in maximizing emotional wellbeing.

CONTINUE GETTING RESTORATIVE SLEEP

Restorative sleep is clearly important for amplifying emotional wellbeing. Please see RESOURCES for CD's focused on getting restorative sleep.

Deep Healing Resources

The emotions of grief and loss typically occur during the cancer journey, particularly when death is the expected outcome. The above suggestions are very practical and extremely effective when dealing with these emotions. In addition, I have written the next section in this book (Section 6) for anyone interested in learning about deep emotional healing. This type of healing deals with your emotional health at a much deeper level. The exercises are more intangible and require a greater investment of time, energy, and emotion, but the results last longer and are more comprehensive, affecting every area of your life in a positive way.

Summary

Sometimes, no matter what weapons we use, cancer wins the battle for our body. And when we know that further fighting is useless, we will deal with grief—there is no way around it. It is a necessary, normal emotional process humans must go through when facing the end of our life. It is also one of the most difficult.

In addition, your loved ones are also grieving. They're grieving their loss of you, while watching you self grieve, while still working hard to "be there for you." It's a difficult time for everyone.

Just like there's no one "right way" to go through cancer, there's no one "right way" to go through grief. But being on the lookout for signs of clinical depression and other over-the-top emotions is advised. Several self-care tools for managing your emotions during this time were shared in this section. Self-care will continue to help you cope as you go through this part of the journey.

In Section 5 we focused on the emotions of grief and loss as they relate to dying and death—for both the cancer patient as well as their loved ones. Numerous tools for coping with these emotions were shared.

Note:

1. "When a Loved One Dies: Coping through a Time of Grief,"
http://www.dignitymemorial.com/en-us/library/article/
name/guidance-series-when-a-loved-one-dies

SECTION 6

EMOTIONAL WELLNESS AND EMPOWERED LIVING

Life is not the way it's supposed to be. It's the way it is. The way you cope with it is what makes the difference.

Virginia Satir

Cancer is a forever chapter in your life.

Regardless of where you find yourself right now—with cancer or without—you won't ever erase how cancer affected you in the past or is affecting you now.

Each of the earlier sections in this book focused on a particular part of the cancer journey such as diagnosis, treatment, recurrence, etc. Specific tools were given for both the patient and the family members to effectively move through it with emotional wellbeing. In each section, a specific emotion was examined and numerous coping tools were shared.

Cancer is intertwined with roller coaster emotions and, therefore, no one emotion is exclusive to a particular part of the cancer journey. You will want to turn to the section that focuses on whichever emotion you're dealing with to see what tools can be most effective for you to use at any given time.

This section is focused on a deeper perspective of emotional wellness. It requires tremendous self-examination for the purposes of discovering clarity and joining it with resilience to connect with emotional wellbeing. That connection is dynamic, demanding a continual shape-shifting of self.

The exploration of emotional wellbeing is much like a buffet—you choose what resonates with you and leave the rest behind. You may find other "foods" to add that aren't discussed here. There is no one right way to attain emotional wellness. It's completely about what makes sense to you and what works for you.

Your Core: Who Are You?

What a strange question to ask. Who are you? You may have known before cancer, but now your answers may be different. Does cancer inspire new answers?

Ask yourself, who am I? I am.............

The truth is you have your core self, the *you* you were before cancer, the *you* you are now with the current experience of cancer, and the *you* you'll be after cancer. That core self doesn't go away.

Your core may feel like it goes away sometimes or that parts of you have gone away. But cancer doesn't have that kind of power—not ever—to take your essence—your core—away from you.

Now, who are you? See if you can answer with clear and confident answers. Write them down. Say them aloud, slowly and firmly. Return to your answers as needed. Yes I am.... It's essential for you to be firmly grounded in who you are.

Niki Barr, Ph.D.

Your Spiritual, Physical and Emotional Self: Who Are You?

Unlike your core (the very essence of you), your spiritual, physical and emotional self changes over your lifetime. As you grow and develop, you naturally add new thoughts and beliefs, discarding those that no longer seem to work. Unsurprisingly, once cancer has been diagnosed, wherever you find yourself in the journey, all three of these may significantly change, or one of them, or some combination of them.

These changes are important to consider.

Who are you now spiritually? I am....

Who are you now physically? I am....

Who are you now emotionally? I am....

As you did in the discussion about your core, write your answers down. Take plenty of time with this exercise. Reflect. Add. Subtract. Leave it for a couple of days and see if your answers change. Read them again in a week, a month, several months.

Knowing where you are with each of these makes it easier to connect and stay connected to emotional wellness. Continue to ask yourself and write down your answers throughout your lifetime.

What lies behind this exercise is that when you know where you stand within your spiritual, physical, and emotional self, you can use that knowledge to help you determine how you will handle whatever life situation you're facing.

203

For example:

Spiritually you're committed to the idea that there is something bigger than humans, whatever you choose to call him/her, and on the whole, life is good, people are good.

Coming from your spirituality, your boss is really tough to deal with, expecting you to do more than you think is possible. Before cancer you liked your work and excelled in it, despite your thoughts about your boss. But now, after cancer, you're very aware of how your boss treats you and others, noticing she likes to keep things stirred up, using subtle intimidation.

You think she's truly a good person and wants the best, but you see that the drama factor doesn't fit with how you believe people ought to be treated. Evaluating your work situation, you decide to begin the process of exploring other work opportunities.

Your physical self doesn't apply to your particular work situation.

Emotionally you like to stay calm and usually do. You learned tools going through cancer to help you effectively get through fear, depression, and overwhelm.

Coming from your emotions, you realize working with a boss that stirs up emotions sprinkled with subtle intimidation doesn't fit for you anymore. You want to work for a boss who is supportive and inspires good work.

Using your spiritual, emotional, and physical self provides a compass for moving through whatever situation you're facing with confident emotional wellness. This is true even though your answers within each of the three may change. The key is knowing where you stand spiritually, emotionally, and physically.

Exploring acceptance of cancer is necessary to further strengthen where you stand spiritually, emotionally, and physically. After reading the next section, Acceptance, come back to this one for possible tweaking.

Acceptance

Acceptance is saying:

- Yes, cancer happened.
- You have cancer.
- You are now cancer-free.
- You're a caregiver or you aren't any longer.

It's easy to say, "Accept what happened." But no one else is in your skin. No one knows exactly what this experience is for you or has been for you or will continue to be for you.

In my professional opinion, acceptance is fundamental for moving your life forward. When you choose not to accept that cancer is/was your reality, you stay caught up in it, much like spinning in circles on a merry-go-round.

But that doesn't mean acceptance is easy.

Acceptance is a process that unfolds on its own. You don't get a map for how to reach acceptance, and sometimes acceptance can come and go depending on your emotions, your current situation, etc.

Acceptance requires spending time with yourself and/or with a therapist, friend, religious leader, etc., sorting through what is happening and what has happened. This undertaking doesn't require you to like it, but it does require you to come to know, within your heart of hearts, that cancer is part of your life experience—however awful, worrisome, stressful, overwhelming, terrifying it is/was. Cancer is what happened.

Then ask yourself, *Now What?* And start moving on to an empowered life.

Now what?

A better question is what do **you** want empowered living to be?

What are your thoughts, hopes, and dreams? These may or may not be different than before cancer.

Be clear with yourself. This isn't about wishing you didn't have to get surgery, or wishing you didn't have chemo brain, or wishing you could work at the same place you did before cancer but can't now because of physical changes. It's not about wishing your loved one didn't have cancer. This is about your life situation as it is right now. What are your thoughts, hopes, and dreams?

Write them down. Then add others to the list. It's a good idea to focus on your list, to daydream about your thoughts, hopes, and dreams, to focus on them, to meditate on them, and to speak about them to those who will be supportive and encouraging.

Look back at the previous topic and think again about your spiritual, physical, and emotional self. What are your dreams for each of those? Continue to explore your answers focused on whatever your situation is right now—just as it is.

Sometimes you don't know what your thoughts, hopes, and dreams are and other times you're very sure. The next section offers suggestions for freeing yourself to move forward toward what you want and provides tools to help you get there.

Freeing Up Energy and Tools to Move You Forward

Dumping Old Baggage

Think of an old suitcase—one you've kept and used forever. The green lining is ripping at the corners and a few brown stains are scattered here and there. The outside is rough, too. The heavy duty material is clearly wearing and strings are sticking out from its stitching. But you hold on to it because you've always traveled with this bag, and it's comfortable, and you don't want to spend money to buy a new one, and....

Here's the problem. You and everyone else carry old history that no longer serves you and, in reality, gets in your way. That argument you had with your sister so long ago you don't even remember when or how it started—it still sits in your craw when you think about it. Or there's your old boss who chose someone else to promote when you know you were the right one for that position, after all you gave to that company. Or it's the ex-spouse who took you for your money. She never loved you for you.

Whatever it is, it's over and done with. Keeping it active hurts you and takes up needed life energy. Find a way to let it go. See a therapist, talk with a friend, or talk with your religious leader. Do something to move past it.

Forgiveness

Forgive yourself for whatever you've done, not done, wish

you had done, should have done, could have done, or would have done. Then forgive everyone else. Forgiving is a huge, necessary part of freeing yourself.

Most people go through a lifetime holding on to hurts that keep on hurting, fueled by their refusal to forgive. Be a forgiver. Pride yourself on forgiving.

What needs to be forgiven? What can you do right now to forgive it?

Guilt

Guilt is powerful, holding you in its tight grip. Beating yourself up never works. It doesn't dispel guilt.

Survival guilt may be swirling round and round in your thoughts. You wonder how did you live and she didn't? How is it you have Stage 1 and they have Stage 111? How is it you had a good scan report and he didn't? But there are no answers.

Working with a therapist can be especially helpful when dealing with guilt. As very difficult as it is for you, somehow being able to let go of guilt and/or survivor guilt is necessary for freeing yourself.

Expectations

You expect he will call, she will do what she said, the surgery will go well, your energy will come back...a zillion things. Carrying expectations is normal. When you have expectations, and we all do, and when they're not met, emotions erupt...anger, frustration, disappointment, confusion, etc. How could you? What were you thinking? Why didn't you?

Why did that happen? Why didn't it happen? What the heck?

Perhaps something better, instead of expectations, is to decide, "We'll see how it unfolds." This way you let yourself and the other person off the hook. Life is dynamic. Nothing can be guaranteed, least of all expectations.

Remember the old story about the farmer.

> A farmer had one horse to plow his fields. One day the horse ran away.
>
> The townspeople said, "That's just terrible. How will you plow your fields?"
>
> The farmer said, "We'll see."
>
> The next day several wild horses stopped to eat leftover hay in the farmer's field and he was able to catch one.
>
> The townspeople were so happy. "You're lucky. Now you have a new horse to plow your fields."
>
> The farmer said, "We'll see."
>
> The farmer's son decided to go for a ride on the new horse, but fell and broke his leg.
>
> The townspeople said, "Oh, that's awful. Now your son can't help you with the farm."
>
> The farmer said, "We'll see."
>
> Then the army came by to recruit the farmer's son, but his leg was broken, so they went on to the next farm.

The townspeople said, "You're so lucky, Your son broke his leg, now he doesn't have to go into the army."

The farmer said, "We'll see."

Expectations are the opposite of allowing things to unfold however they will. Life does the unfolding anyway, despite our desires and demands. Consider more "unfolding" and less expectation.

Gratitude

Everyone talks about it and many of us are indeed both grateful and thankful. Could you step it up and be even more so?

When your thoughts and words speak of gratitude, you're free to focus on what is working, what is good, what you like, what you appreciate. A gratitude focus, when it's genuine, keeps your mind free from what ties you down.

Fear

Fear is something that is just there with cancer. The key is managing your fear. When you're caught up in fear, instead of trying to push it down, look at it. Have a conversation with it. Something like:

> *"What's going on?"*
>
> *"What specifically am I afraid of?"*
>
> *"Do I need to take any action about this fear?" (Possibly see the doctor or schedule a therapist appointment?)*
>
> *"It's ok to feel afraid."*

"On a scale from 1-10, with 10 being highest fear, where am I?"

"What could I do to move one number down?" (And then another.)

Work with your fear. Feeling afraid of your fear makes it grow. Having a conversation with it is actually soothing and validates the emotion.

Do this for all your emotions. Trying to wish them away never works for any length of time.

Dreams

I've had many people tell me in psychotherapy of intense dreams about cancer. Often they're repetitive and tend to be frightening. That's normal. It's part of how you're working through all that has happened and is happening. I encourage you to talk with a therapist who can help you sort through your dreams. You also may want to keep a journal of them.

If you can, look at dreams as serving you, helping you move forward. What can you learn from them?

Passing of Time and Patience

You may now have a sense of urgency about time. Others around you don't necessarily feel it, but you do. Cancer changes how you feel about time.

Additionally, your sense of feeling patient may change. Before cancer, you felt more casual about things getting done or maybe you've always been impatient. Once cancer comes into the picture, it's not unusual to feel less patient.

Relationships

Relationships become hugely important after cancer comes. Those you thought would be there for you aren't necessarily, and those you didn't have a clue would show up, do.

You may also find yourself pulling back from relationships, needing a lot more space alone. That's okay. Just take action if you notice you're getting depressed in a way that's interfering with your daily functioning.

One of the most difficult phases is when you've completed medical treatment and your family and friends expect life to go on as if nothing happened. You wonder how this is possible. Life has forever changed for you. You cannot just ignore what's happened.

You'd like them to acknowledge and validate that you've moved through cancer. You'd like them to ask a simple question—How are you? Really, how are you? You'd like them not to trip over the white elephant in the living room and not to expect that you've totally wiped cancer out of your memory forever.

Have a heart-to-heart chat with them, but be prepared that your friends probably still don't get it. Take note—that's not about you. Rather, it speaks loudly about them and their discomfort around cancer. But it's difficult not to take it personally.

And think through your friendships. You may need to weed some out because they no longer support and nourish you. It's okay to do this.

Meditation

Many people meditate and many people say, "I just don't get it. That's not for me. I can't," etc.

Meditation is very useful for clearing your mind of pesky thoughts that won't leave you alone. It's good for receiving intuition since you've quieted yourself to hear it. It's also good for significantly decreasing stress.

Different ways to meditate can be found everywhere. If you don't meditate, you may want to try just sitting quietly in a chair by yourself without distraction. Just sit there, close your eyes, and "be." If thoughts come, don't engage with them, just let them come. If your phone rings, let it ring. If the doorbell rings, let it ring. If you get a text, let it be.

The idea is to be quiet, if only for a few minutes. Meditation is much like a muscle, the more you do it, the easier it becomes.

Refuse to get caught up with, "I don't know how." There is no magic about meditation. There's not an exact right way. You find your way. A good start is by carving out time every day, preferably in the morning before life takes off, to just be still.

Consider the "Re's"

According to the online English Oxford Dictionary, "Re" is a prefix meaning "once more, afresh, anew."

Afresh and anew particularly apply to you, given the cancer roller coaster ride you've been on. Consider these words and how you can use them to help you move from "a fresh" and "a new" perspective. With your life situation as it is now (surgery still needed, chemo brain, no evidence of cancer, active

caregiver), how do you use the following words/tools to ac-
tualize what you want for yourself.

Re-balance: spiritual, physical, and emotional

Re-create: what you want

Re-envision: now

Re-do

"Re-see"

"Re-hear"

Re-invent

Re-juvenate

Re-lease

Re-solve

Re-store

Re-shape

Re-fine

Re-vamp

Re-order

Re-call

Re-bound

EMPOWERED DAILY LIVING WITH EMOTIONAL WELLBEING

Self-care, self-compassion, and self-respect are necessities that help you live in an empowered way. Life before cancer may or may not have included these, but life after cancer must include these. Before cancer maybe you didn't think about or have time for self-care, self-compassion, and self-kindness, but now these three take top priority for empowered living.

Self-care is defined as spending time doing what you love. Identify those things and make certain you get self-care every day. Self-care recharges you for handling whatever is on your agenda.

In the past, self-care was noted as the last item on your to-do list, if it even made your list at all. Self-care in our society was—and sometimes still is—considered selfish. How are you to take care of anything else in life if you're not taking care of you? Much like a car must have fuel to run, you must have energy to work with. Self-care provides energy.

Self-compassion is defined simply as having compassion for yourself. It's forgiving yourself when you didn't do what you set out to do, or you didn't say the "right" thing, or other similar situations. You've never lived this exact experience before, so give yourself a break. Keep in mind how you'd treat your best friend, then do that for yourself.

Self-respect means being respectful of yourself. When you're tired, see that you get more sleep. When you have a conflict with someone, talk about it with her/him. When you need a break, take one. Honor your own self. Many people have said you teach people how to treat you. Yes, you do. And the foundation is how you treat yourself—or self-respect.

Intention

Setting an intention for what you want is a big deal. Many ignore this. But keeping your focus on your hopes and dreams for yourself matters greatly. Every morning set an intention for how you'd like the day to go, and for how you'll move forward on realizing your desires.

Take Your Pulse

In order to keep yourself on course, develop a habit of checking in with yourself.

> *How am I doing?*

> *What am I feeling?*

> *What do I want/need right now?*

Think about driving a car. When you drive, you're constantly correcting with little movements. As the road turns you move the wheel to stay on it. When your destination requires turning right, you turn right.

Pay attention to the little adjustments you need to make throughout your day in order to keep moving forward.

Use this same tool to check in with yourself spiritually, physically, and emotionally, taking actions to keep you on course with your desires.

> *Spiritually, how am I doing? What am I feeling? What do I want/need right now?*

> *Physically, how am I doing? What am I feeling? What do I want/need right now?*

Emotionally, how am I doing? What am I feeling? What do I want/need right now?

Write Love Letters to Yourself

Living is not easy for anyone. Never in my lifetime have I met someone who said, "Oh, everything in my life is perfect all of the time." That's not the nature of life on earth.

Once cancer comes into your life, everything is at least a thousand times more complicated, regardless of what you're going through or have gone through.

No one knows what it's like for you personally, even if you've shared intimate details. Only you know what it's like living in your own skin. Therefore, you must look after yourself and your own emotional wellbeing.

A wonderful way to do this is to write notes and letters of encouragement to yourself. This isn't the time to worry what someone else will think. Who cares? This life is about you, moving you forward to realize your hopes and dreams for yourself, even though cancer is/was part of your life experience. This life is about you moving forward with yourself exactly as you are now, with life exactly as it is now.

Be bold and write a note! Here are a couple of examples.

Dear Me,

Thank you. Thank you for moving forward even when you didn't feel like it, even when you didn't get the support you wanted, even when you were very scared, confused, and overwhelmed. I appre-

ciate me and I'm grateful I have me to live my life.

I love you!
Love Me

Dear Me,

I can't believe that person just said that. What was she thinking? I'm so sorry you had to hear that. She clearly doesn't get it. I choose not to take what she said inside of me.

I love you!
Love, Me

Dear Me,

Maybe instead of expecting so much from myself, I could just give myself a break. It's okay. I'm doing everything I can right now. I don't have to know how everything will unfold, because I can't. What I can do is live five minutes at a time, continually taking good care of myself.

I love you!
Love, Me

This may be a new—really new—experience for you. We aren't taught to write nice notes to ourselves. But why wouldn't you do this? It's one little way to encourage yourself to keep moving forward.

Resilience

Much is written about resilience these days because resilience is required for making it through the challenges of daily life. Add cancer to that life and resilience becomes absolutely essential for moving forward.

The definition of resilience according to the Merriam-Webster online dictionary is:

> "The ability to become strong, healthy, or successful again after something bad happens."

> "The ability of something to return to its original shape after it has been pulled, stretched, pressed, bent, etc."

But that's not my definition of resilience. My definition is taking yourself where you are right now and going on in the best way you can, treating yourself with compassion, kindness, and respect.

You get there through resilience. If you misspell resilience, you get there through
re-silence.

Re-silence yourself. Come inward to your core, to your spirit, body, and emotion. Celebrate that rawness of who you are and celebrate it with every single breath you take. You do this for you. That's what's important.

Re-silencing yourself through meditation or through quiet thought brings you what you need to go forward, even if it's one minute at a time. Re-silencing brings peace, calm, soothing when there's none to be found around you. Going within brings balance and energy for whatever is next.

Re-silence is the ace in your pocket, your best of best friends, the biggest and most valuable tool in your toolbox. It's the thing that connects you with you. And nothing can touch that—not even cancer.

Summary

Your choice to live an empowered life—in spite of disease—is a testament to your bravery. With all of the changes that continue to affect you, it would be much easier to live a lesser life. This section, like the previous ones, offers a number of tools for you to choose from. But unlike the others, this section primarily focuses on tools that will help you gain insights into yourself.

Empowered living develops from the foundation of self-awareness—awareness of who you really are—in your core and in your spiritual, physical, and emotional self.

Self-care, self-compassion, and self-respect are essential ingredients, combining to propel you and keep you moving forward. Continually taking time to check in with yourself will help you make needed course corrections, and keep you on track—living the empowered life you deserve.

CONCLUSION

THE END IS ONLY EVER THE BEGINNING

There will come a time when you believe everything is finished. That will be the beginning.

Louis L'Amour

Congratulations on exploring and using the tools in this book to help you get off the emotional roller coaster of cancer—even if only for short periods of time. Returning to these tools often, to re-explore and re-use them as needed, will help keep you anchored through life's ups and downs.

I celebrate your commitment to move forward, in spite of a society that doesn't foster checking in, or asking you how you really are, or helping you cope with sometimes paralyzing emotions, or just listening to you—truly listening to you.

I believe every end is a new beginning. So even though this is the end of my book, it can be the beginning of a new way of life for you. You can now use the tools you've acquired here to live an empowered life.

An empowered life continually seems to require restarting, refreshing, and renewing. And a lot of people don't want to invest that much in themselves. Instead they choose to live a lesser life.

What they don't understand is that the only alternative to living an empowered life is to stay stuck.

But you understand.

And it's very clear—you won't be doing that.

RESOURCES

This list is designed as a starting place for your research. New resources are available everyday. You'll want to screen carefully to determine what is helpful and credible and what is not.

Cancer Emotion Tools

Sections 1-5 of this book each focuses on specific emotions that are very prevalent during the cancer journey. Multiple tools are listed and described to help you cope with that particular emotion. However, no one emotion fits neatly in each phase.

Listed here are all the emotions that are covered and where in this book to find the tools to help you cope. Whenever you're dealing with one or more of these emotions, come here for the location of the tools you need to keep moving forward.

Emotion	Section	Tools Begin on Page
Anger	4	153
Anxiety	1	14
Depression	3	110
Grief	5	182
Loss	5	190
Overwhelm	2	59

Books

The Artist's Way. Julia Cameron, 1992, 2002 Penguin Putnam, Inc.

Chicken Soup for the Soul: The Cancer Book: 101 Stories of Courage, Support & Love. Jack Canfield, Mark Victor Hansen and David Tabatsky, 2009 Soul Publishing, LLC

Chicken Soup for the Breast Cancer Survivor's Soul: Stories to Inspire, Support and Heal. Jack Canfield, Mark Victor Hansen and Mary Olsen Kelly, 2012 Soul Publishing, LLC

Crazy Sexy Cancer Survivor: More Rebellion and Fire for Your Healing Journey. Kris Carr, 2008 Skirt! Publishing

Embrace Release Heal. Leigh Fortson, 2011 Sounds True, Inc.

Everything Changes: The Insider's Guide to Cancer in Your 20s and 30s. Kairol Rosenthal, 2009

Getting Past the Fear: A Guide to Help You Mentally Prepare for Chemotherapy. Nancy Stordahl, 2014

Magazines

Cancer Today: http://www.cancertodaymag.org/Pages/default.aspx

Coping with Cancer: http://copingmag.com/cwc/

Cure: http://cur.magserv.com

CD's

Guided Mindfulness Meditation. Jon Kabat-Zin. http://www.mindfulnesscds.com/collections/cds

How to Meditate with Pema Chodron: A Practical Guide to Making Friends with Your Mind. Pema Chodron http://www.dharmacrafts.com/9FRG/2084CD/how-to-meditate.html?gclid=CMmH1YnJs78CFUYA7AodIG4Axw

Just Relax- Relaxing to Sleep CD. Gail Seymour http://www.justrelax.cc/benefits.htm

Meditation for Beginners. Jack Kornfield http://www.jackkornfield.com/audiosets/#Meditation%20for%20Beginners

Meditation to Help You with Healthful Sleep. Belle Ruth Naparstek http://amandawashington.blogdetik.com/2014/02/10/health-journeys-a-meditation-to-help-you-with-healthful-sleep-by-belleruth-naparstek/

Meditation For Relaxation. Niki Barr, PhD http://canceremotionalwellbeing.com/order/

Meditation For Soothing Anxiety. Niki Barr, PhD http://canceremotionalwellbeing.com/order/

Sleep Through Insomnia. KRS Edstrom http://www.healthjourneys.com/Store/Products/Sleep-Through-Insomnia/282

Websites

Advance Directives. http://www.caringinfo.org/i4a/pages/index.cfm?pageid=3289

American Cancer Society. http://www.cancer.org

Breastless in the City: A Young Woman's Story of Love, Loss, and Breast Cancer. http://cathybueti.com/breastlessinthec-itysynopsis.asp

Cancer Support Community. http://www.cancersupportcom-munity.org

Cancer.Net. Oncologist-approved cancer information from the American Society of Clinical Oncology. http://www.cancer.net/

Complementary and Alternative Medicines. nccam.nih.gov/sites/nccam.nih.gov/

Empathy vs. Sympathy Video. http://www.openculture.com/2013/12/the-power-of-empathy.html

LiveStrong. http://www.livestrong.org

National Cancer Institute. http://www.cancer.gov

National Coalition for Cancer Survivorship. http://www.can-ceradvocacy.org

Planet Cancer. http://myplanet.planetcancer.org/Planet Cancer

Stupid Cancer: The Voice of Young Adult Cancer. http://stu-pidcancer.org/

"Would You Date a Cancer Survivor?" (Article on Curetoday. com) – This lists some on-line dating/friendship sites specif-ically for cancer patients. http://www.curetoday.com/index.cfm/fuseaction/blog.showIndex/laceymeyer/2009/7/20/Cancer-and-dating--online

Young Survival Coalition. – a wonderful organization specifically for young women with breast cancer...I posted a message on their forum requesting advice about when to tell my date about cancer, and their responses were thoughtful and detailed. I highly recommend the site to any young woman with breast cancer (and her friends and caregivers). http://www.youngsurvival.org/

About the Author

Niki Barr, Ph.D., founded a pioneering psychotherapy practice dedicated to working with cancer patients in all stages of cancer, as well as with the patient's spouse or partner, children, family members, caregivers, and friends.

In *Getting Off the Emotional Roller Coaster of Cancer* she shares the many insights, strategies, and tools she has discovered while working with thousands of cancer patients over the course of her practice.

Dr. Barr is a dynamic and popular speaker in clinics and hospitals, at workshops, seminars and conferences, speaking on the subject of "Emotional Wellbeing Within Cancer." In addition to audiences of cancer patients, family members, caregivers and friends, Dr. Barr often speaks to professionals establishing or refining their counseling skills within the oncology field.

Niki loves being in her garden, growing organic fruits and vegetables, then creating wonderful meals from them. When she's not outside or in the kitchen, she's knitting. Niki and her husband live in the Dallas area with their dog, Miss Tilly.

For more information about Dr. Barr, her practice, and her media calendar, visit her website, www.CancerEmotionalWellness.com. You can also connect with her via:

Facebook: www.facebook.com/CancerEmotionalWellBeing

Twitter: @NikiBarrPhD

LinkedIn: Niki Barr, Ph.D.

YouTube: Niki Barr, Ph.D.

Google+: Niki Barr, Ph.D.

Made in the USA
San Bernardino, CA
27 October 2014